Frontiers in Boron-based
Medicinal Chemistry

Other Titles by the Editor

Fundamentals and Applications of Boron Chemistry

Boron and Gadolinium Neutron Capture Therapy for Cancer Treatment

Frontiers in Boron-based Medicinal Chemistry

Editor

Yinghuai Zhu

HEC Pharm Co. Ltd., China

World Scientific

EW JERSEY · LONDON · SINGAPORE · BEIJING · SHANGHAI · HONG KONG · TAIPEI · CHENNAI · TOKYO

Published by

World Scientific Publishing Co. Pte. Ltd.

5 Toh Tuck Link, Singapore 596224

USA office: 27 Warren Street, Suite 401-402, Hackensack, NJ 07601

UK office: 57 Shelton Street, Covent Garden, London WC2H 9HE

Library of Congress Cataloging-in-Publication Data
Names: Zhu, Yinghuai, editor.
Title: Frontiers in boron-based medicinal chemistry / editor Yinghuai Zhu.
Description: New Jersey : World Scientific, [2023] | Includes bibliographical references and index.
Identifiers: LCCN 2022058929 | ISBN 9789811267963 (hardcover) |
    ISBN 9789811268038 (ebook) | ISBN 9789811268045 (ebook other)
Subjects: LCSH: Boron-neutron capture therapy. | Pharmaceutical chemistry.
Classification: LCC RC271.R3 F758 2023 | DDC 615.1/9--dc23/eng/20230414
LC record available at https://lccn.loc.gov/2022058929

British Library Cataloguing-in-Publication Data
A catalogue record for this book is available from the British Library.

For any available supplementary material, please visit
https://www.worldscientific.com/worldscibooks/10.1142/13191#t=suppl

Desk Editor: Shaun Tan Yi Jie

Typeset by Stallion Press
Email: enquiries@stallionpress.com

Preface

Boron is an electron-deficient element, so boron-containing drugs generally have an electrophilic center at boron and tend to accept lone pair electrons from nucleophiles such as enzymes and proteins. After accepting a lone pair of electrons, the boron atom changes from an sp^2 hybrid with trigonal conformation towards an sp^3 hybrid which has tetrahedral conformation. The unique chemistry of boron-based drugs has thus attracted broad interest from both academia and industry.

This book describes advanced boron-based drugs, applications and related pharmacology based on the authors' collective and latest research results. It details general boron chemistry, FDA-approved boron-containing drugs, as well as emerging boron agents, theranostics, neutron sources and clinical reports for boron neutron capture therapy. The basis of the design, development and potential pharmaceutical applications of the relative boron compounds is emphasized in each chapter. From the contents, the reader can study and/or refresh the general principles and unique characteristics of boron-based medicinal chemistry, be updated with developments in the applications of boron-containing drugs, and hopefully initiate creative ideas in the field. Therefore, this is a very useful guide for undergraduate and postgraduate students of chemistry and their instructors, researchers in medicinal and inorganic chemistry, as well as practitioners and professionals in the pharmaceutical industry.

Figures where a reference number is indicated at the end of the caption are reproduced from published works, with kind permission from the respective publishers.

Yinghuai Zhu
Singapore, October 2022

About the Editor

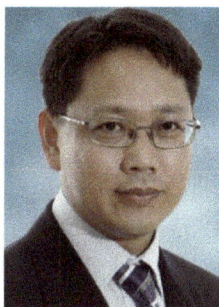

Dr. Yinghuai Zhu is Expert Scientist at HEC Pharm Co. Ltd., China. He was previously Senior Scientist for 15 years at Agency for Science, Technology and Research (A*STAR), Singapore. He was also Associate Professor at Macau University of Science and Technology and Nankai University, China, as well as Visiting Scientist at Northern Illinois University, USA. His research focuses on boron chemistry and catalysis. He has published over 100 articles in top peer-reviewed journals, and edited the books *Boron and Gadolinium Neutron Capture Therapy for Cancer Treatment* and *Fundamentals and Applications of Boron Chemistry*.

Contents

Contents

꽃

Chapter 1

General Boron Chemistry and Medicinal Applications

Yinghuai Zhu

Sunshine Lake Pharma Co. Ltd., China

Abstract

Boron is a unique element with electron-deficient properties. In nature, it appears as boric acid and inorganic borates rather than in elemental form. Boron chemistry has been well developed, and a tremendous amount of new boron-containing compounds and materials have been reported. Consequently, boron has found a wide range of applications in fine chemistry, material science, new energy generation and drug development. In particular, boron-based small molecule drugs have attracted enormous attention in recent decades, of which some have been approved by the FDA for clinical use. As a result, boron-containing compounds have been employed in both chemotherapy and radiotherapy to treat different types of patients. Naturally, boron has two main isotopes, boron-11 and boron-10. Boron-10 is capable of absorbing thermal neutrons and initiating a nuclear fission reaction. The reaction generates and releases linear high-energy alpha (α) particles that can destroy tumor cells, so the concept has been utilized in boron neutron capture therapy and nuclear power plants, to treat cancer patients and reduce neutron leakage, respectively. Since the book aims to update and analyze advances in boron-based medicinal chemistry, this chapter first introduces basic boron chemistry and provides a brief overview of the clinical applications and perspectives of organoboron compounds typically involved in disease treatments.

Keywords: neutron capture therapy, boron chemistry, carborane, boron drug, anti-cancer drug, anti-tuberculosis, anti-malaria drug, neglected tropical disease.

1.1 Elemental Boron

On the periodic table, the chemical element boron is located in group 13 and period 2 with an electronic configuration of $1s^2 2s^2 2p^1$. According to the octet rule, six electrons are usually required to be placed in the p-orbital to form a stable valence shell of total eight electrons ($2s^2 2p^6$). Therefore, elemental boron is electron-deficient due to its lack of an octet of electrons. Consequently, boron compounds are usually also electron-deficient and thus recognized and employed as strong Lewis acids which may readily react with Lewis bases, which have electron-pair donors, to form corresponding adducts.

Boron is capable of forming stable covalent bonds either by an sp^2 or sp^3 hybrid. The covalently bonded molecular networks of boron may demonstrate several amorphous and crystalline forms [1]. Crystalline boron shows high physical and chemical stability. Its melting point is greater than 2000°C. Three crystalline allotropes of boron have been discovered, namely the α-rhombohedral (α-R), β-rhombohedral (β-R), and β-tetragonal (β-T) [1]. Two naturally occuring, stable isotopes of boron are known, ^{11}B (80.1%) and ^{10}B (19.9%). Due to its extremely high neutron cross section, the ^{10}B isotope is commonly used in capturing thermal neutrons in the nuclear industry [2].

In boron chemistry, boron usually adopts an sp^2 hybridization when forming new chemical bonds, and that leads to the formation of a planar, triangular boron compound. Obviously, the compound is electron-deficient due to a retaining empty p orbital, and can act as a Lewis acid to accept free electrons of an electron-rich group such as a Lewis base to form an sp^3 hybrid tetrahedral complex. In case there are no additional electrons available, self-polymerization can occur to form the electron-deficient multi-center bonds, such as three-center

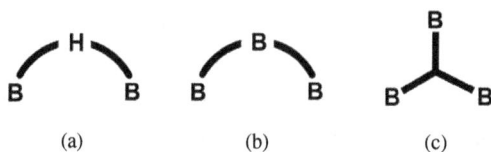

Figure 1.1   Electron-deficient multi-center bonds of boron: (a) hydrogen bridge bond, (b) boron bridge bond and (c) three-center two electron boron bond.

two-electron hydrogen bridge bonds, three-center two-electron boron bridge bonds and three-center two-electron boron bonds as shown in Figure 1.1. The multi-center bond plays a decisive role in the stability and electronic properties of the molecular system.

1.2 General Boron Chemistry

Boron is recognized as the smallest of semi-metals in the periodic table; it hybrids both metal and non-metal properties. Boron can form oxides such as B_2O_3 and salts such as $B_2(SO_4)_3$ that behave like metals. When forming acids such as H_3BO_3, boron demonstrates non-metal chemical properties. As mentioned above, boron atoms are trivalent with vacant p-orbitals, which make most of the borocompounds electron deficient. By adopting a hybrid of sp^2 or sp^3, boron binds with a few elements such as groups 6 and 7 elements in the periodic table, to form either a triangular planar or tetrahedral structure, respectively.

The trigonal planar molecular structures are usually extremely reactive in aqueous solution compared to the tetrahedral species, which are chemically very stable and, consequently, stabilize polymer linkages or participate in a chemical catalytic process. In comparison with stable crystalline boron, amorphous boron is relatively reactive. It slowly reacts with oxygen in air to form the boron trioxide at room temperature; the rate of oxidation depends on the crystallinity, particle size, purity and temperature. When heated to around 700°C, boron ignites spontaneously with a red flame, and a green flame when vaporized [1,3]. Even though pure boron is aqueous insoluble, it reacts with both concentrated acids such as concentrated nitric acid and concentrated sulfuric acid, as well as aqueous base solutions such as sodium hydroxide solution as shown in Eqs. (1.1)–(1.3). When heated, boron reacts with water vapor to generate boron hydroxide and release hydrogen (Eq. (1.4)). Under elevated temperature, pure boron is capable of reacting with many non-metals, metals and metal oxides to form metal borides. For example, boron and sulfur react violently to form boron sulfide at about 600°C; when boron is heated in nitrogen or ammonia above 1000°C, boron nitride can be formed; boron and silicon react above 2000°C to produce silicon boride. The resulting advanced metal boride materials usually show extreme hardness, high conductivity, melting resistance and chemical inertness [1,3].

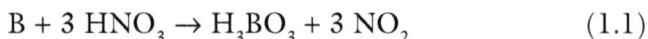

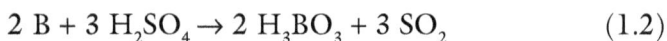

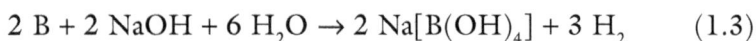

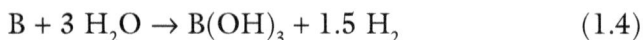

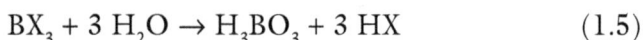

$$B + 3\ HNO_3 \rightarrow H_3BO_3 + 3\ NO_2 \qquad (1.1)$$

$$2\ B + 3\ H_2SO_4 \rightarrow 2\ H_3BO_3 + 3\ SO_2 \qquad (1.2)$$

$$2\ B + 2\ NaOH + 6\ H_2O \rightarrow 2\ Na[B(OH)_4] + 3\ H_2 \qquad (1.3)$$

$$B + 3\ H_2O \rightarrow B(OH)_3 + 1.5\ H_2 \qquad (1.4)$$

$$BX_3 + 3\ H_2O \rightarrow H_3BO_3 + 3\ HX \qquad (1.5)$$

Boron is an oxyphilic element, meaning it can extract oxygen from many stable oxides such as water and silicon oxide to form boron oxides, and thus boron can be used as a reducing agent [1–4]. Directly burning crystalline boron at high temperature forms boron trioxide. Boron trihalides are additionally frequently used boron compounds, both in fine chemistry and in the pharmaceutical industry. Boron adopts the sp^2 hybridization in the trihalides with a trigonal planar structure. Boron trihalides are also Lewis acids, and react with electron-pair donors (also called Lewis bases) to readily form stable adducts. On the other hand, boron hybridization may also change in the trihalides from sp^2 to sp^3. For example, boron trifluoride (BF_3) reacts with fluoride (F^-) to generate the tetrafluoroborate anion, $[BF_4]^-$. Boron trifluoride is commonly used in the petrochemical industry as a catalyst and as a convenient boron source in organic synthesis. The boron halides are found to violently hydrolyze to form boric acid as shown in Eq. (1.5) [1–3].

1.3 The Preparation of Elemental Boron

Four existing approaches are available to prepare elemental boron: hydrogen reduction of the boron halide, metal thermal reduction, molten salt electrolysis and thermal decomposition.

(1) **Halide hydrogen reduction method.** At a temperature of 1200–1400°C, the mixed gas of boron trihalide and hydrogen passes through a tungsten or tantalum wire, the boron trihalide is reduced and produces elemental boron forming a sheet or needle-like structure on the wire. This method prepares the elemental boron with a high purity of up to 99.999% (Eq. (1.6)) [1–3].

$$2\ BX_3 + 3\ H_2 \rightarrow 2\ B + 6\ HX\ (X = Cl,\ Br) \qquad (1.6)$$

(2) **Metal thermal reduction method.** In this method, boric acid, boron oxide, fluoroborate, and borohydride are used as the boron sources, while metals and/or semi-metals such as lithium, sodium, magnesium and silicon are used as the reducing agents [1–3]. Among the metals, magnesium is often used to reduce boric acid or boron trioxide (Eq. (1.7)). The process is also used in the industry to prepare elemental boron, as presented in Scheme 1.1. Here, the boron source is first decomposed with concentrated sodium hydroxide to form and crystallize sodium metaborate, which is dissolved in water to form its more concentrated solution. In the following step, the alkalinity is neutralized by adjusting with carbon dioxide to crystallize and separate the borax product after concentration. The borax is then dissolved in water and the acidity

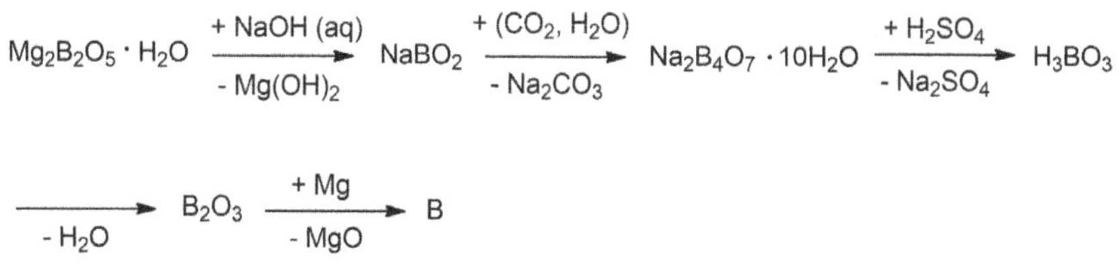

$$Mg_2B_2O_5 \cdot H_2O \xrightarrow[- Mg(OH)_2]{+\ NaOH\ (aq)} NaBO_2 \xrightarrow[- Na_2CO_3]{+\ (CO_2,\ H_2O)} Na_2B_4O_7 \cdot 10H_2O \xrightarrow[- Na_2SO_4]{+\ H_2SO_4} H_3BO_3$$

$$\xrightarrow[- H_2O]{} B_2O_3 \xrightarrow[- MgO]{+\ Mg} B$$

Scheme 1.1 The production of elemental boron in the industry.

adjusted with sulfuric acid to precipitate boric acid crystals due to its lower solubility. After heating boric acid, a dehydration reaction occurs to produce boron trioxide. Eventually, the boron trioxide is reduced with metals such as magnesium and aluminum to generate crude boron. By treating the crude boron with hydrochloric acid, sodium hydroxide and hydrogen fluoride in sequence, amorphous boron can be obtained with a purity of 95–98%.

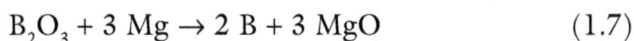

$$B_2O_3 + 3\ Mg \rightarrow 2\ B + 3\ MgO \qquad (1.7)$$

(3) **Molten salt electrolysis method.** Three types of molten salt systems, (a) B_2O_3-KCl, (b) KBF_4-KCl, and (c) KBF_4-KF-KCl or KBF_4-KCl-NaCl have been investigated to prepare elemental boron by electrolysis [1–3]. A boron carbide anode is used for electrolysis. However, the method obtains low purity of the elemental boron, generally at the level of 87–99.8%.

(4) **Thermal decomposition method.** The reduction materials used in the thermal decomposition process are limited to halide and borohydride, such as boron bromide and diborane, respectively. The decomposition reactions are usually conducted at a temperature range of 1073–1773K. High-purity boron can be prepared by this method [1–3]. In the laboratory, elemental boron has also been prepared by thermal decomposition reactions. For example, the pyrolysis of a decaborane ($B_{10}H_{14}$) cluster forms boron nanoparticles at a high temperature range of 973–1173K in an inert atmosphere [5]. Recently, Zhu *et al.* reported that boron isocyanates could be reduced to generate boron nanoparticles under a mild condition of 1 atm (hydrogen) at 323K [6]. The resulting boron nanoparticles could be chemically functionalized for further applications [7].

1.4 Boron Compounds with Important Influence

1.4.1 *Boranes*

Borane is a generic name used to describe compounds being composed mainly of boron and hydrogen (B_xH_y). Most common known boranes include borane (BH_3), diborane(6) (B_2H_6), pentaborane(9) (B_5H_9), decaborane(14) ($B_{10}H_{14}$), decaborate(10) anion ($[B_{10}H_{10}]^{2-}$), dodecaborate(12) anion ($[B_{12}H_{12}]^{2-}$) and octadecaborane(22) ($B_{18}H_{22}$). In these non-classically bonded compounds, each boron atom is directly connected with a hydrogen atom to construct a polyhedral molecular scaffold. The multi-center bonds decide both the stability and electronic properties of the molecular system. The following multi-center bonds explained by William Lipscomb, among others, are involved within these molecules: B–H–B bonds (3-center-2-elctron), B–B–B bonds (3-center-2-electron), and B–B, B–H bonds (2-center-2-electron) [9]. William Lipscomb made special efforts on studying the molecular structures of boranes, for which he won the Nobel Prize in Chemistry in 1976 [9]. In addition, the structures of boranes can also be well predicted with Wade's rules, also known as the polyhedral skeletal electron pair theory [10]. In general, the structures of boranes are classified as *closo*-type ($[B_nH_n]^{2-}$, *e.g.*, $[B_{12}H_{12}]^{2-}$), *nido*-type (B_nH_{n+4}, *e.g.*, B_5H_9, $B_{10}H_{14}$) and *arachno*-type (B_nH_{n+6}, *e.g.*, B_4H_{10}) polyhydroboranes as shown in Figure 1.2.

The simplest borane, trihydridoboron (BH_3), has three valence electrons. Therefore, boranes are Lewis acidic, and tend to accept free electron pairs. Trihydridoboron is prepared by a reaction between boron trihalide (BX_3 (X = F, Cl, Br, I)) and a borohydride anion ($[BH_4]^-$) [3]. Two molecules of BH_3 form diborane (B_2H_6) *via* a

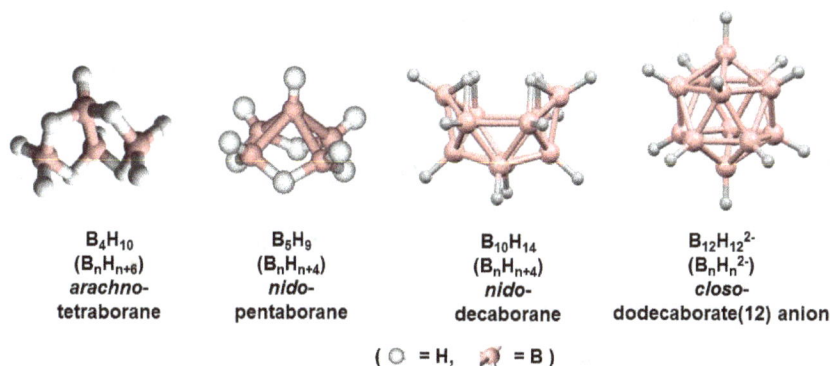

B_4H_{10}	B_5H_9	$B_{10}H_{14}$	$B_{12}H_{12}^{2-}$
(B_nH_{n+6})	(B_nH_{n+4})	(B_nH_{n+4})	($B_nH_n^{2-}$)
arachno-	*nido*-	*nido*-	*closo*-
tetraborane	pentaborane	decaborane	dodecaborate(12) anion

(○ = H, ◆ = B)

Figure 1.2   Representative examples of polyhydroboranes.

7

self-conjugation reaction. In addition, BH_3 is capable of adducting with other Lewis bases (L) such as diethyl ether, tetrahydrofuran and dimethyl sulfide to form the thermodynamically stable compounds ($L \cdot BH_3$). Among these structures, the Lewis base donates its lone pair of electrons to the electron-deficient boron center to form a coordinate covalent bond. In the industry, diborane is produced by reducing BF_3 with a metal hydride donor such as NaH and LiH as shown in Eq. (1.8) [11]. However, for a small-scale production in the laboratory, reductants $LiAlH_4$ and $NaBH_4$ are commonly used. In addition, oxidation of a borohydride salt also is used in a laboratory preparation of diborane together with iodine in diglyme as solvent [11].

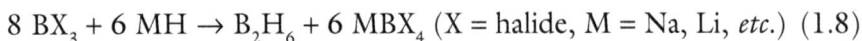

$$8\ BX_3 + 6\ MH \rightarrow B_2H_6 + 6\ MBX_4\ (X = \text{halide}, M = \text{Na, Li, } etc.) \quad (1.8)$$

Small boranes such as BH_3 and B_2H_6 are extremely reactive. They are flammable in air and react with oxygen to generate boron trioxide and water. They also can react with water and alcohols to yield boric acid and trialkyloxyborate ester, respectively, while releasing hydrogen gas [11]. Importantly, small boranes have been widely used in organic synthesis as hydroboration reagents; they perform the hydroboration of alkenes and alkynes. The addition reaction follows high regioselectivity to obtain the less substituted alcohol after further oxidation and hydrolysis reactions. In that procedure, hydrogen peroxide and aqueous sodium hydroxide are commonly used to treat the borane adduct intermediates. The adduction is recognized to follow a so-called "anti-Markovnikov" selectivity, and the resulting new OH and H are *syn* to each other in the alcohol product (Eq. (1.9)) [12,13].

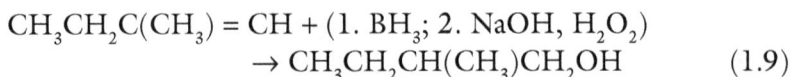

$$CH_3CH_2C(CH_3) = CH + (1.\ BH_3; 2.\ NaOH, H_2O_2)$$
$$\rightarrow CH_3CH_2CH(CH_3)CH_2OH \quad (1.9)$$

Decaborane(14) (*nido*-$B_{10}H_{14}$) is another principal borane (Figure 1.2). Decaborane(14) is a white crystalline solid with a strong foul odor, and is highly flammable, toxic and volatile. Therefore, it can be purified by sublimation, similar to naphthalene [14]. Decaborane(14) is prepared either by the pyrolysis of smaller boranes such as diborane

(B_2H_6) and pentaborane (B_5H_9) [15], or by a process designed by Dunks *et al.* in which the diethyl ether adduct of boron trifluoride $(BF_3 \cdot OEt_2)$ reacts with sodium borohydride $(NaBH_4)$ to form an intermediate, $NaB_{11}H_{14}$, which is worked up with aqueous sulfuric acid to give the desired crude product in a yield of around 40% [16]. The proposed overall reaction is summarized in Eq. (1.10). However, the small borane gases used in the pyrolysis processes are hazardous and explosive, which make them hard to handle and which require relatively elaborate manufacturing facilities. Therefore, the method of Dunks and coworkers is preferred in laboratory preparations of decaborane(14).

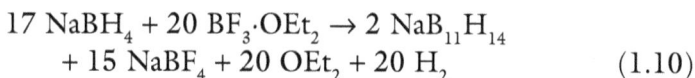

$$17 \, NaBH_4 + 20 \, BF_3 \cdot OEt_2 \rightarrow 2 \, NaB_{11}H_{14}$$
$$+ \, 15 \, NaBF_4 + 20 \, OEt_2 + 20 \, H_2 \qquad (1.10)$$

Decaborane(14) has a *nido*-framework resembling an incomplete octadecahedron. It reacts with varying substrates such as Lewis bases to give so-called *arachno* adducts [14]. These *arachno* clusters can react with a carbon-carbon triple bond to give various *closo*-carboranes as shown in Scheme 1.2. Therefore, decaborane(14) has been used as an important precursor to prepare other boron hydride clusters and carboranes. Carboranes have found wide applications in coordination chemistry to form various metal complexes. Nevertheless, few other applications have been reported for decaborane(14) due to its relatively high toxicity in affecting the central nervous system and high explosivity.

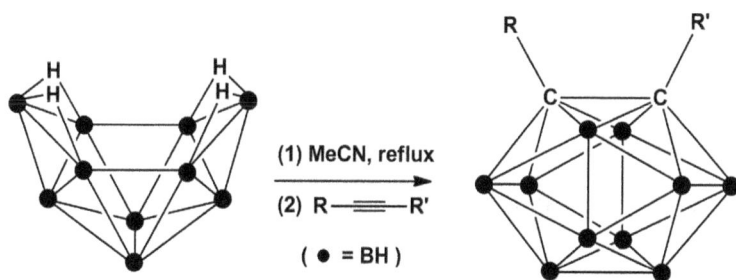

Scheme 1.2 Synthesis of *closo-ortho*-carboranes from decaborane(14).

1.4.2 Boronic Acids

Boronic acids, $RB(OH)_2$, are important members of organoboranes, and have been extensively used in fine chemistry as a building block to form new carbon-carbon bonds by reacting with an aryl halide counterpart. Usually catalyzed by a palladium-based complex, it is well known as the Suzuki cross-coupling reaction [17]. Boronic acids are also Lewis acids due to their electron-deficient boron centers, and thus also can react with Lewis base donors such as alcohols and amines to form conjugating adducts. Some adducts are reversible covalent complexes when the Lewis base has 1,2 or 1,3 donors. This phenomenon has been observed and used in the life sciences to elucidate the pharmacodynamics of boron-containing drugs and *in vivo* glucose examination technology.

Currently, three main types of methods are commonly used to prepare various boronic acids, described as follows and shown in Scheme 1.3 [17].

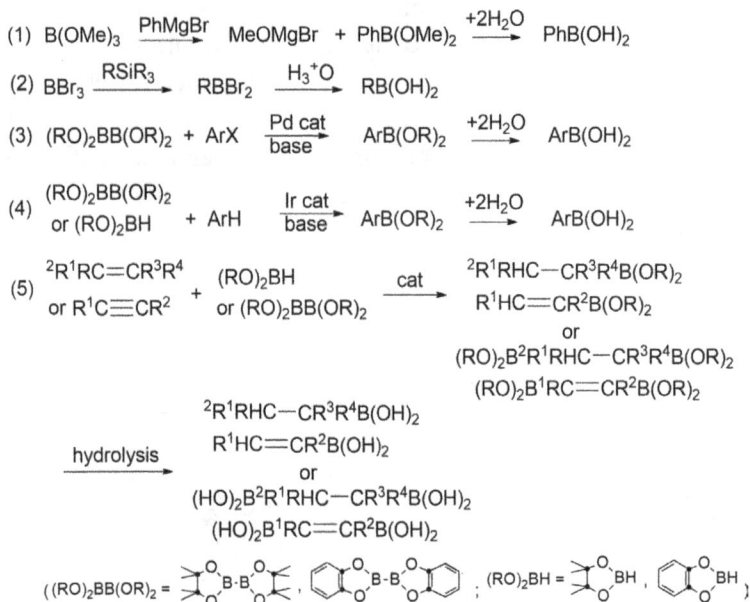

Scheme 1.3 Methods used to synthesize boronic acids.

(1) In the first method, trimethyl borate reacts with a Grignard reagent derived from phenylbromide to give a phenylborate intermediate, which undergoes hydrolysis to produce phenylboronic acid. In the process, other borate esters such as tributyl borate and Grignard reagents such as phenyllithium may also be used as starting materials depending on the individual reactions.

(2) Alternatively, a boron halide such as boron tribromide is treated with an arylsilane to form an arylboron dibromide intermediate *via* a transmetallation reaction. The intermediate can further react with an aqueous acid to give the boronic acid product.

(3) A third method is a catalytic conversion process, which is much safer, environmentally benign, and convenient to handle. It is well known as the Miyaura borylation reaction [18], where a palladium-based catalyst and base are commonly used in the reaction. Besides diborate, tetrahydroxydiboron, $(HO)_2BB(OH)_2$, is also used as a boron source [17,18].

(4) In addition, a fourth method, known as a C–B coupling reaction, has emerged and been developed in the last two decades [19–23]. In this reaction, a carbon-hydrogen bond reacts directly with a boron compound, such as bis(pinacolato)diboron and pinacolborane, to form an aromatic boronate. The aromatic boronate can further undergo hydrolysis reaction to give the boronic acid. The transition metal complex-based catalysts such as $IrCl(cod)_2$ (cod=1,5-cyclooctadiene) [22,23] and $Cp*Rh(\eta^4-C_6Me_6)$ [24], and organobases such as substituted bipyridine, are commonly used in the method. Alkanes have also been reported to undergo similar catalytic borylation reactions to form the alkyl borates or boronic acids [24,25].

(5) Finally, the borane or diborane is capable of reacting with an unsaturated carbon-carbon double or triple bond to form the corresponding borylated adduct. Similar to other borylation methods, the boronic acids may be obtained *via* hydrolysis of the parent precursors [26–28].

Boronic acids are widely used in organic synthesis to form new chemical bonds such as carbon-carbon and carbon-nitrogen bonds, and hence have been playing crucial roles in the medicinal industry such as the preparation of drugs. Among the C–C coupling reactions, the Suzuki–Miyaura cross-coupling reaction [29–31], Petasis boronic acid–Mannich reaction [32,33] and Roush asymmetric allylation reaction [34–38] have been well developed and commonly used. In the Suzuki reaction, as shown in Scheme 1.4, a halide compound including alkyl, alkenyl or aryl halide reacts with an organoboronic acid to form a new C–C single bond [29–31,39,40]. Besides organohalides, vinyl thioethers and amides are also capable of undergoing a C–C cross coupling

Suzuki-Miyaura cross-coupling reaction

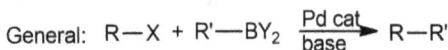

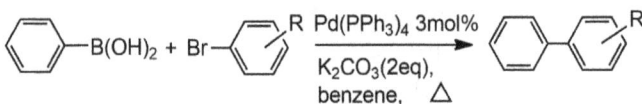

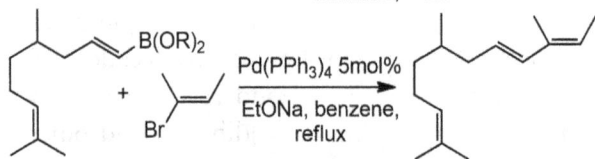

Petasis boronic acid-Mannich reaction

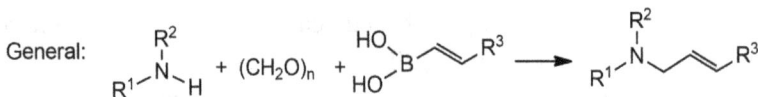

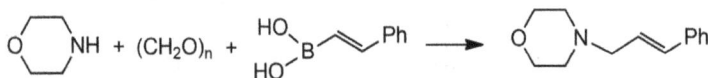

Roush asymmetric allylation reaction

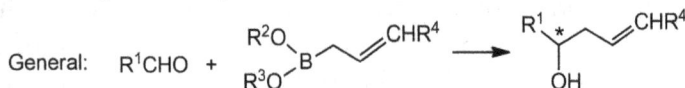

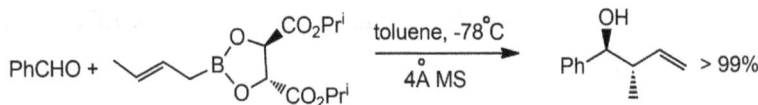

Scheme 1.4 Representative examples of C–C coupling reactions using organoboronic acids.

reaction with the borate. For example, it has been reported that multi-substituted olefins and conjugate dienes were synthesized with regio- and stereoselectivity by using alpha-oxo ketene dithioacetals as the building blocks [41]. The reaction is proposed to proceed *via* a palladium-based catalytic cycle. In the amide coupling reactions, nickel-based catalysts can be used to construct the new C–C bonds (Eq. (1.11)) [42].

Boronic acids are widely used in C–C coupling reactions due to their wide variety and they are a comparatively cheaper resource, being commercially available. However, boronic acids tend to undergo a well-known undesired side reaction: protodeboronation [43]. The protonolysis is frequently associated with transition metal-catalyzed C–C coupling. Nevertheless, the propensity for the reaction is highly connected to various factors such as molecular structure and reaction conditions used. Therefore, other organoboranes such as aryltrifluoroborate are also employed in the Suzuki cross-coupling reaction, because they are less prone to protodeboronation compared to boronic acids [44]. Briefly, an aryl boronic acid reacts with potassium hydrogen fluoride (KHF_2) leading to the formation of the aryltrifluoroborate, which subsequently undergoes the cross-coupling (Eqs. (1.12) and (1.13), respectively) [45]. In addition, the Suzuki cross-coupling reaction has been further developed to improve its atom economy and environmental benefit, with greener solvents such as water and ionic liquids employed in the procedure [46].

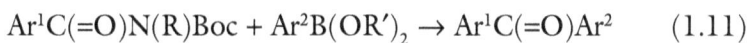

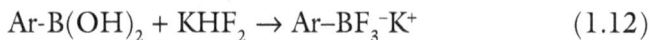

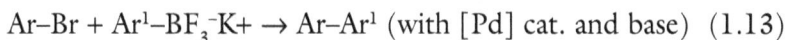

$$Ar^1C(=O)N(R)Boc + Ar^2B(OR')_2 \rightarrow Ar^1C(=O)Ar^2 \quad (1.11)$$

$$Ar\text{-}B(OH)_2 + KHF_2 \rightarrow Ar\text{-}BF_3^-K^+ \quad (1.12)$$

$$Ar\text{-}Br + Ar^1\text{-}BF_3^-K+ \rightarrow Ar\text{-}Ar^1 \text{ (with [Pd] cat. and base)} \quad (1.13)$$

In the Petasis boronic acid-Mannich reaction, a vinyl boronic acid reacts with an amine and paraformaldehyde to form an allylamine (Scheme 1.4). Here, the boronic acid works as a nucleophile and paraformaldehyde participates as a carbon source [32,33]. In 1985, Roush *et al.* reported that chiral allylic boronates react with achiral aldehydes to give homoallylic alcohols with high yield and enantioselectivity (Scheme 1.4) [34–38]. The reaction, known as Roush asymmetric allylation, has been developed and substrate scope has been extended widely. The approach was used for total synthesis of the anticancer topsentolide B2 diastereomers [38].

Boronic acids have also been employed to form a new carbon-nitrogen or carbon-oxygen bond. In the coupling reaction, the organoboronic acid reacts with a compound containing an N–H or O–H bond in the presence of a copper-based catalyst [47,48] as shown in Scheme 1.5. In addition, Bhanage and coworkers reported an efficient approach to synthesize tertiary amides from aryl boronic acids and inert tertiary amines [49]. The reaction was proposed as a palladium-catalyzed oxidative carbonylation *via* a carbon-nitrogen bond activation (Scheme 1.5). The study complements and develops the synthetic methodologies of amides together with previous works [50–53]. However, the reaction conditions suffer from disadvantages of high CO pressure, limited substrate scope, long reaction time and relatively low yield for aliphatic secondary amines. Moreover, aryl boronic acids have lower nucleophilicity, therefore high dissociation energy and selective functionalization are also required to initiate the oxidative carbonylation reactions.

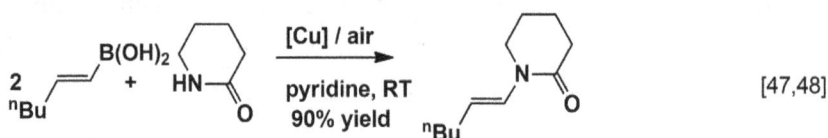

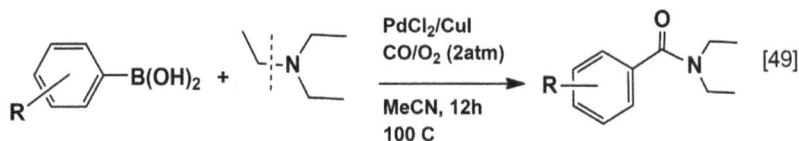

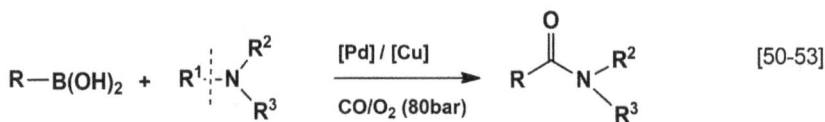

Scheme 1.5 Strategies for amide synthesis through aminocarbonylation.

1.4.3 *Carboranes*

Carborane is a kind of cluster in which one or more carbon atom(s) is/ are presented as an integral part of an electron-delocalized borane framework. The carboranes are a new class of compounds distinct from other organoboron species such as the abovementioned arylboranes and alkylboranes, in which the carbon is presented as a ligand rather than as the cage itself. In principle, carboranes could be conveniently considered as derivatives of the boron hydrides in which boron anions or BH groups are replaced by isoelectronic carbon atoms. The theory of structure and bonding in the boranes, which was developed by Lipscomb and others, plays fundamental roles in carborane chemistry [54,55]. The fact that boron possesses only three valence electrons forced recognition that the bonding in these compounds could not be precisely analogous to that in the hydrocarbons. This so-called "electron deficiency" raised formidable difficulties in dealing with the bonding in the boranes, and in the absence of unequivocal structural data the problem initially remained unsolved. A series of neutral $C_2B_{n-2}H_n$ carborane cages was suggested, each one formally derived from its isoelectronic $B_nH_n^{2-}$ analog by replacement of two B^- with two C atoms. Most of these cage molecules are relatively stable thermodynamically, some of them extremely so, and available chemical and physical evidence strongly suggests that substantial electron delocalization is responsible for their stability. In the carboranes, it is significant that the carbon atoms participate in the delocalized bonding. Therefore, the usual empirical rules of coordination and valency in general organic chemistry are irrelevant to these structures. For example, in $C_2B_{10}H_{12}$, each carbon atom is hexacoordinate [56].

Carborane chemistry is complicated, with the existence of carbon reaction sites in the cluster enabling a versatile and extensive derivative chemistry. For instance, it has been reported that transition metals and heteroatoms (such as Fe and P, respectively) can be bound to the carborane skeleton [57]. Like boranes, carborane clusters are classified as *closo-*, *nido-*, *arachno-*, *hypho-*structures, *etc.* They are defined as *closo-*carborane when they represent a completely closed polyhedron structure. When one, two or three vertices are missing, the structures are called *nido-*, *arachno-* and *hypho-*carborane, respectively. Further categorization can be made according to the position of the carbon atoms in the cluster. For example, $C_2B_{10}H_{12}$ can be classified as 1,2-, 1,7- and 1,12-$C_2B_{10}H_{12}$. They are also known informally as *ortho*-carborane, *meta*-carborane and *para*-carborane, respectively, as shown in Figure 1.3 [57]. When heated at a high temperature of 475–600°C, the *ortho*-isomer may convert to the *meta*-isomer by a thermal rearrangement process. The *meta*-carborane undergoes the similar thermal rearrangement to give the *para*-isomer at high temperatures of 650–700°C [58]. All the three isomers are commercially available.

The *ortho*-carborane is chemically more active in comparison with the *meta*- and *para*-isomers. It is prepared in high yield by reaction of the decaborane-Lewis base complex $(B_{10}H_{12}L_2)$ with acetylene [59]. The use of substituted acetylenes consequently results in C-substituted *closo*-carborane derivatives. The *ortho*-carborane cage is relatively stable and demonstrates resistance to degradation when compared to the boranes. The *ortho*-carborane unit displays strong electron-withdrawing character with respect to substituents attached at the carbon atoms. This property is reflected, for example, in the ease of metalation of the *o*-carborane C–H group, the strong acidity of *o*-carborane carboxylic acids, and the relative stability of halomethyl-*o*-carboranes with respect to nucleophilic reagents. In contrast, *meta*-carborane and *para*-carborane are far less electrophilic.

Two general methods are employed to prepare derivatives of *ortho*-carborane substituted at the carbon atoms. One of them is the

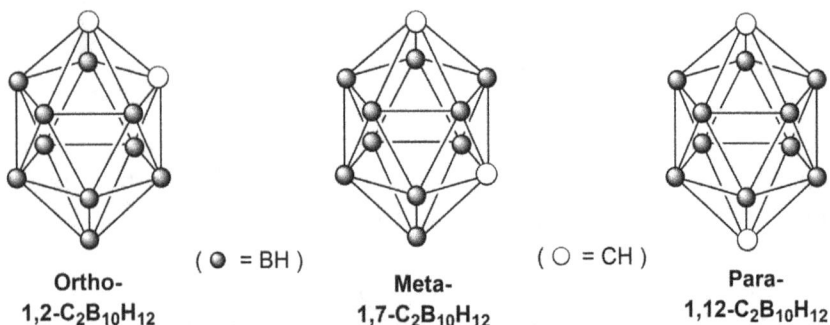

(● = BH) (○ = CH)

Ortho-
1,2-$C_2B_{10}H_{12}$

Meta-
1,7-$C_2B_{10}H_{12}$

Para-
1,12-$C_2B_{10}H_{12}$

Figure 1.3 The isomers of carborane $C_2B_{10}H_{12}$.

metalation of *ortho*-carborane followed by treatment with reagents such as aldehydes, organic and inorganic halides, epoxides and others to form mono- or di-carbon-functionalized *ortho*-carboranes. The mildly acidic C–H bonds in *ortho*-carborane react easily with a suitable base such as *n*-butyllithium, phenyllithium or sodium hydride to form C-lithium (or -sodium) *ortho*-carborane; an excess of the organometallic reagent yields the C,C′-dilithio derivative. The anion intermediate can further conduct a nucleophilic displacement or addition reaction to form mono- or di-carbon-functionalized *ortho*-carboranes. A second approach involves the reaction of substituted acetylenes with bis(ligand) decaborane compounds.

In ether or ether/benzene, but not in benzene itself, an equilibrium exists between the mono- and dilithio species (Figure 1.4). Lithium exchange has also been found in attempts to prepare *ortho*-carboranyl monocarboxylic acid by reaction of the monolithio derivative with carbon dioxide in ether; it yields the dicarboxylic counterpart in addition to the desired monocarboxylic acid. However, in benzene, the monocarboxylic acid is obtained in good yield [60,61]. For the *meta*- and *para*-carborane systems, the equilibrium lies much further to the left, with less than 2% dilithio-carborane in equilibrium with the monolithio species.

Ortho-carborane-based Grignard reagents are formed in reactions of *ortho*-carborane with alkyl magnesium halides and by the reaction of magnesium on 1-halomagnesio-*ortho*-carboranes. The chemistry of the halomagnesio-*ortho*-carboranes is complicated, exhibiting equilibria of the type observed for lithiocarboranes in tetrahydrofuran solvent.

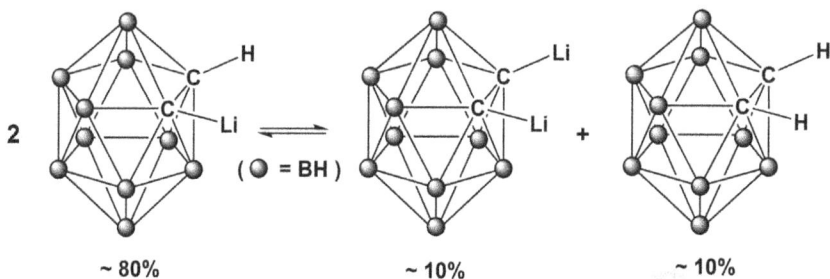

Figure 1.4 The equilibrium of the mono- and dilithiocarborane species.

Consequently, reactions of 1-bromomagnesio-*ortho*-carborane with alkyl halides yield mixtures of mono- and disubstituted carborane products. Reactions of 1-bromomethyl-*ortho*-carboranes with magnesium were expected to give 1-halomagnesiomethyl carborane derivatives. However, it was found that in tetrahydrofuran solvent, rearrangement to 1-methyl-2-bromagnesio-*ortho*-carborane is extensive, as shown in Scheme 1.6. Therefore, carbonation of the Grignard prepared from 1-bromomethyl-*ortho*-carborane in tetrahydrofuran yields 1-methyl-2-carboxylic acid-*ortho*-carborane. However, carbonation of the same Grignard in ether produces mainly *ortho*-carboranyl acetic acid, indicating that rearrangement occurs to a much lower extent in this solvent for C-aryl- and C-alkyl-*ortho*-carboranes. The possibility of rearrangement is eliminated in Grignards having a methyl or other alkyl group on the second *ortho*-carborane carbon atom. Such reagents produce the expected reactions of organomagnesium compounds [56,62].

C-aryl- and C-alkyl-*ortho*-carboranes are conveniently prepared from a bis-ligand decaborane derivative and the appropriate substituted acetylene as described above. The alkynyl and alkenyl carboranes can also be prepared with this approach. For example, vinylacetylene reacts with bisacetonitriledecaborane to produce 1-vinyl-*ortho*-carborane in

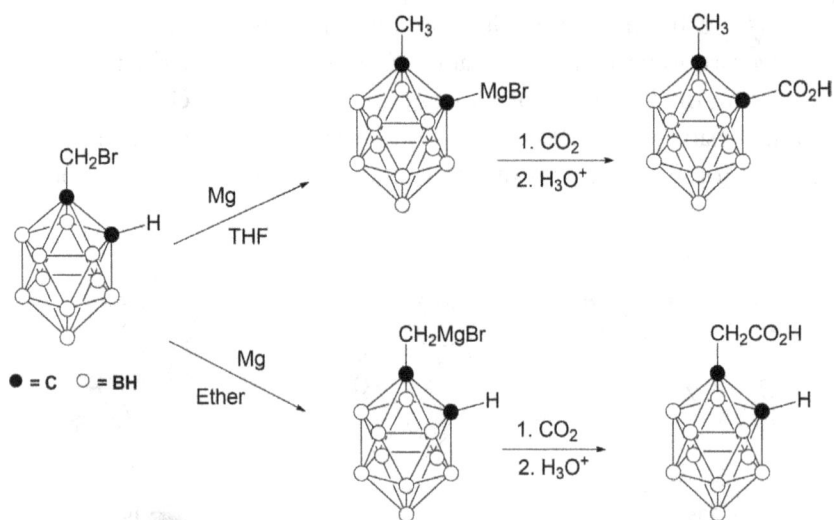

Scheme 1.6 Reactions of 1-bromomethyl-*ortho*-carboranes with magnesium.

high yield. Alternatively, C-aryl- and C-alkyl-*ortho*-carboranes may be prepared *via* reactions of C-metalated derivatives of *ortho*-carborane with primary alkyl bromides or iodides, usually in benzene, ether or liquid ammonia [59] as shown in Scheme 1.7. It should be noted that secondary and tertiary alkyl halides do not react with metallocarboranes, and primary chlorides react only slowly. The method may be used to prepare exocyclic ring derivatives of *ortho*-carboranes from dimetallo-*ortho*-carboranes [59]. The bis(halomagnesium)carboranes react with a,ω-dihaloalkanes to form exocyclic groups such as 1,2-*ortho*-carboranylcyclopentane. In addition, dimetallo-*ortho*-carborane such as $Li_2[C_2B_{10}H_{10}]^{2-}$, which is prepared *via* deprotonation by *n*-BuLi, may react with bromine at 0°C followed by slightly heating the reaction mixture at 35°C to generate carboryne *in situ*. The resulting carboryne can react with an alkyne or diene to give an exocyclic species such as a triptycene-like molecule (from anthracene addition) or a benzocarborane (from alkyne addition) [57].

According to the electrophilic character of the *ortho*-carboranyl system, the following conclusions have been obtained: (1) the *ortho*-carboranyl system is a powerful electron acceptor due to an inductive mechanism, where the strength of the inductive effect is roughly comparable to the halogens; (2) the inductive effect of the *ortho*-carboranyl unit is much weaker when the ligand is attached to B(3) than when the connection is at C(1); (3) the electron-withdrawing tendency of the *meta*-carboranyl system is considerably weaker than that of the *ortho*-carboranyl; (4) there is no appreciable ground-state extension of electron delocalization caused by interaction of an aryl group with the *ortho*-carborane species.

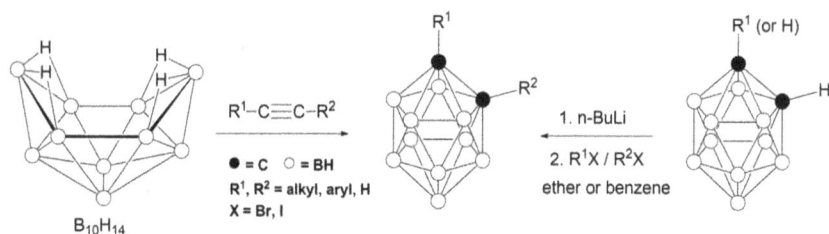

Scheme 1.7   Synthesis of C-aryl- and C-alkyl-*ortho*-carboranes.

When reacting with bases such as inorganic sodium hydroxide or organic pyridine, *ortho*-carboranes undergo decomposition and release one B atom to form *nido*-carboranyl anions. The anions can be further deprotonated to give the corresponding dianion derivatives. The resulting dianion ($[C_2B_9H_{11}]^{2-}$) has been found to be a unique type of coordination ligand which can form various transition metal complexes. It is well recognized that carboranyl dianions are an isolobal analogy of the cyclopentadienyl dianion; they have 6 π electrons delocalized on the C_2B_3 or C_2B_4 open faces of the dianions. The dianions can coordinate metals in an η^5 or η^6 fashion to form corresponding metallocarboranes with either a sandwich or a half-sandwich molecular structure [63]. Due to the similarities, these carborane-based transition metal complexes have been investigated as catalysts for olefin polymerization. It has been found that carboranyl ligand-coordinated complexes, particularly for group 4 compounds, can be active pre-catalysts for olefin polymerization [64]. In particular, half-sandwich metallocenes including bridged cyclopentadienyl and amido ligands, also known as constrained geometry complexes (CGCs), are excellent catalysts for ethylene polymerization [65]. Such complexes were generally prepared *via* the following straightforward method: (1) the *closo*-carborane clusters were deprotonated and functionalized by nucleophilic reactions; (2) the functionalized *closo*-carboranes were decapitated either by MOH (M = Na, K) or alkali metals (Na, K) to form *nido*-carborane anions; (3) the resulting *nido*-carboranes underwent metalation to give the carborane-based CGCs. Various π-coordinated metallocarborane-based CGCs have been reported so far (Figure 1.5) [64]. They are inherently thermally and chemically stable. They also show advantages of tunable electronic and steric effects of the carboranyl ligands, and therefore are potentially promising and structurally unique pre-catalysts. However, these catalysts usually show low to moderate activity compared to the existing Dow CGC catalyst. It is necessary to modify both functional groups attached to carborane cages as well as the metal center to develop high active catalysts for olefin polymerization. Other applications of these carboranyl metal complexes are also being explored in fine chemical and pharmaceutical processes.

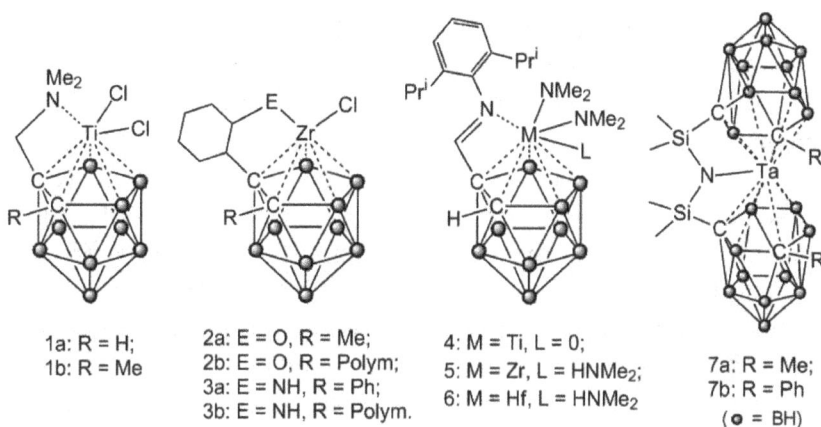

1a: R = H;
1b: R = Me

2a: E = O, R = Me;
2b: E = O, R = Polym;
3a: E = NH, R = Ph;
3b: E = NH, R = Polym.

4: M = Ti, L = 0;
5: M = Zr, L = HNMe2;
6: M = Hf, L = HNMe2

7a: R = Me;
7b: R = Ph
(● = BH)

Figure 1.5 π-Bonded carborane-based CGC catalysts for ethylene polymerization [64].

The *meta*-carborane chemistry is less explored in comparison. However, the reactions and properties of *meta*-carboranes parallel those of *ortho*-carboranes to a considerable extent. For instance, *meta*-carborane is also easily metalated at the carbon atom of the cluster, and results in the formation of metallo-*meta*-carboranes, which are convenient precursors to a large number of C-substituted carboranes. However, *meta*-carboranes are generally weaker electron attracting and more thermally stable. The derivatives of meta-carboranes are less polar, more volatile, and with lower melting point compared to their *ortho*-carborane analogs. The *ortho*-carboranyl species possess high electron affinities, and are more easily reduced. Finally, the *para*-carborane remains rare due to limited production in the decomposition of *meta*- or *ortho*-carborane at a high temperature of above 600°C. Nonetheless, with an improved approach of continuous process to produce *para*-carborane, the chemistry of the species could be extensively developed [66].

1.5 Boron Compounds for Pharmaceutical Applications

1.5.1 *Boron-containing Drugs Approved by the FDA*

As previously mentioned, due to electronic deficiency of the boron atom, boron compounds are often electrophiles, also known as Lewis acids. They tend to accept free electrons from a Lewis base to fill their empty p-orbital, and consequently conduct an interconversion from the trigonal sp^2 to the tetrahedral sp^3 hybridization state. This association is recognized as the principal module of organoboron compound-based enzyme inhibitors, and thus numerous boron-containing bioactive molecules have been developed accordingly [67,68]. Figure 1.6 shows some commonly used organoboron compounds approved by the FDA for clinical use. Bortezomib, 1, developed by Takeda Pharmaceutical, was approved by the FDA in 2003 for the clinical treatment of multiple myeloma [69]. It is a dipeptide of corresponding boronic acid precursors. Tavaborole, 2 (5-fluorobenzoxaborole), was approved by the FDA in 2014 for the treatment of onychomycosis [70,71], and Ixazomib, 3, in November 2015 for the treatment of patients with multiple myeloma in combination with lenalidomide and dexamethasone [72]. Crisaborole, 4, another benzoxaborole, was approved in 2016 for clinical use in the treatment of mild-to-moderate atopic dermatitis [73]. In the U.S. market, it is traded under the name of EUCRISA®. Currently, it is the first and only non-steroidal in anti-inflammatory monotherapy as the phosphodiesterase type 4 inhibitor, commonly referred to as a PDE4 inhibitor for the skin. Compound 5, trade name Vabomere®, was approved in 2017. It is indicated for the treatment of patients with complicated urinary tract infections caused by susceptible bacteria [74]. Vabomere is administered by vein injection. To reduce the development of drug-resistant bacteria and maintain the effectiveness of Vabomere and other drugs, it is strongly recommended that Vabomere should be used alone to treat or prevent infections. It has been found that benzoxaboroles possess unique physical and chemical properties, such as low toxicity, excellent chemical stability, ease in synthesis, and high targeting specificity. These characteristics make them very attractive therapeutic drugs [75].

It is well recognized that the current treatments for tropical diseases are sub-optimal, and in some cases, there are no drugs available to date. Furthermore, drug resistance for the clinically used antibiotics and anti-protozoan agents remains one of the world's serious public health problems. On the other hand, organoboron compounds show high potential in the treatment of cryptosporidiosis and toxoplasmosis [76].

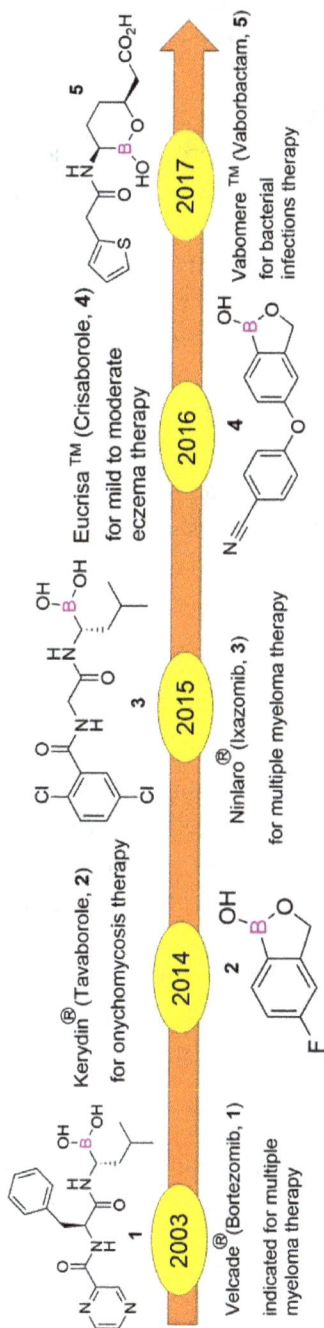

Figure 1.6 FDA-approved boron compound drugs.

Cryptosporidiosis is caused by *Cryptosporidium parvum*, with high morbidity in developing countries [77,78], while toxoplasmosis is caused by infection of the *Toxoplasma gondii* parasite, which has different types of life cycles [79]. It has been found that aminoacyl-tRNA synthetases play essential roles in protein synthesis, therefore they are suitable targets for antimicrobial drug design for parasitic diseases [80]. Various benzoxaborole compounds were designed according to the strategy, and examined as new agents against *Cryptosporidium parvum* and *Toxoplasma gondii* to discover new potential drugs. Compounds 3-aminomethyl benzoxaboroles (AN6426) and its 4-bromo analogue (AN8432) were found to be active candidates. The activities were comparable to that of nitazoxanide, which is the current standard of care for the treatment of cryptosporidiosis [81]. Results were also consistent with that of AN6426-inhibited protein synthesis in both *Cryptosporidium* and *Toxoplasma* by forming a covalent adduct with tRNALeu [81]. Therefore, benzoxaboroles targeting Apicomplexan parasites warrant further development.

1.5.2 *Boron-containing Drugs for Boron Neutron Capture Therapy (BNCT)*

BNCT is a radiotherapeutic modality based on nuclear capture that occurs when non-radioactive, stable ^{10}B isotope is irradiated with low energy neutrons (< 0.5 eV) [82–90]. After hitting a slow neutron, ^{10}B converts to an excited state of the ^{11}B isotope which quickly decays, producing high-linear energy transfer α particles (^{4}He, helium-4) and recoiling lithium-7 nuclei (^{7}Li) (Figure 1.7a). These induce the ionization and excitation of biologically essential molecules, such as proteins, RNA and DNA, within 10 µm, about equal to the size of a single cell, restricting the BNCT impact to boron-accumulating tumor cells without interference to normal cells. And, if the ^{10}B-containing molecules are accumulated preferentially within a tumor cell, the irradiation of the tumor area provides selective destruction of the malignant cells.

In order to be successful in BNCT treatment, an adequate amount of ^{10}B and thermal neutrons must be adsorbed to have killing effects on

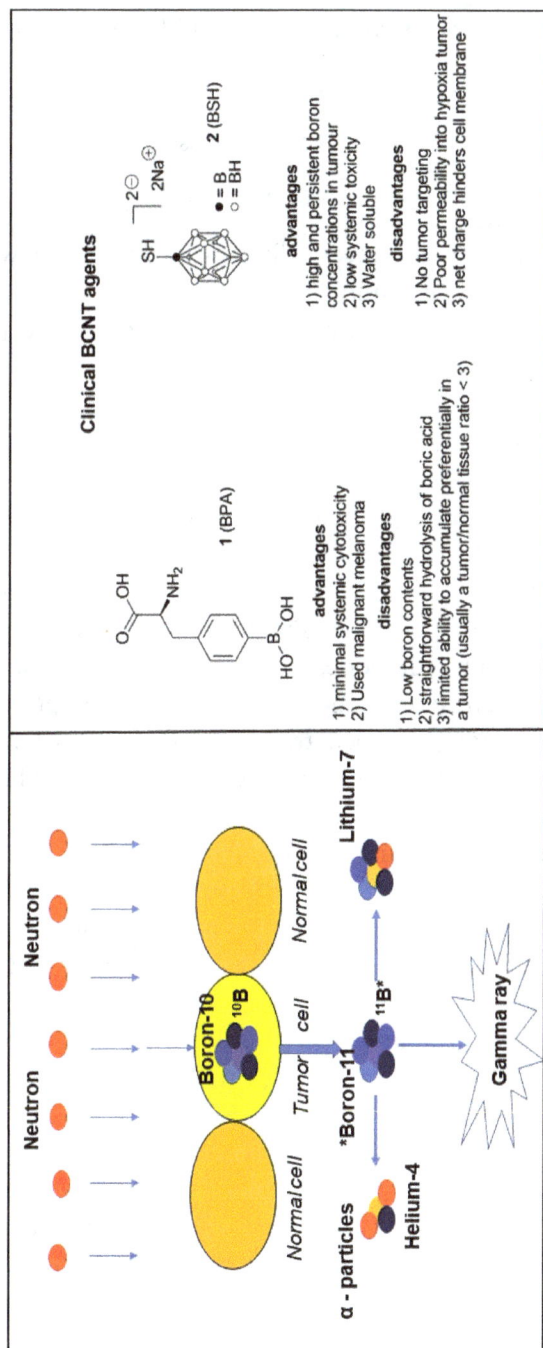

(a)

(b)

Figure 1.7 (a) The principles of boron neutron capture therapy (BNCT); (b) Chemical structures and characteristics of p-boro-L-phenylalanine (**1**, L-BPA) and sodium borocaptate (**2**, BSH).

tumor cells. Moreover, boron compounds should meet the following requirements:

- Rapid clearance from blood and normal tissues than from tumor during BNCT;
- Low systemic toxicity;
- Retention time of boron in cancer cells must be at least a few hours;
- Constant concentration in tumor during BNCT;
- High tumor/normal tissue (T/N > 5) and tumor/blood (T/B > 3.5) concentration ratios;
- High tumor uptblake, 20–50 µg/g of ^{10}B;
- Moderate water solubility.

The first boron-containing molecules used for clinical trials of BNCT during the 1950s–1960s included boric acid (H_3BO_3), sodium tetraborate and their derivatives because of their lack of cytotoxicity, availability and known pharmacology. Preliminary tests were performed on malignant gliomas but with modest outcomes of therapeutic efficacy on all forms of treatment due to the usage of boron compounds that lack selectivity and inadequate penetration of the thermal neutrons [91,92]. Following these limited results, studies conducted by Hatanaka gave rise to fresh interest in BNCT and led to the discovery of a second generation of boron compounds [93]. Among them, the boron-containing amino acid, (L)-4-dihydroxy-borylphenylalanine 1 (BPA, boropharan-^{10}B, Figure 1.7b) [94] and boron cluster with mercapto moiety, sodium mercapto-*closo*-undecahydro-dodecaborate 2 (BSH, $Na_2B_{12}H_{11}SH$, sodium borocaptate, Figure 1.7b) have received clinical attention [95]. Based on amino acid 1, BPA-fructose complex was designed, a water-soluble derivative used in BNCT to treat patients with high-grade intracranial gliomas since 1994 [96].

Nevertheless, the two drugs show inherent disadvantages such as relatively low bio-selectivity of tumor to blood and sparing water solubility of pristine BPA. Although conjugating with fructose may improve the water solubility of BPA, significant amounts of BPA-fructose complex are used clinically, which may be harmful to patients. According to the results of pharmacological studies, it is suggested that BPA may be selectively delivered to malignant cells by L-type amino acid transporters (LAT), such as LAT1 and $ATB^{0,+}$ (amino acid transporter $B^{0,+}$) [97]. However, the localization and mRNA/protein expression of these transporters are tissue dependent in humans, and that may partially result in significant variability of boron uptake for individual patient and specific tumor [98]. Besides the difference in amount and location of the transporter expressions, complex intratumorally genomic and histologic heterogeneity could also contribute to the variability in BPA uptake by tumor cells [97,98].

On the other hand, BSH is a *closo*-dodecaborate, ionic compound with high boron content, high water solubility and low toxicity. BSH was found to accumulate to a very low extent in brain, bone, muscle and fat tissue, but to a high degree in liver and kidney [99]. Although currently BSH adsorption and metabolism remain unclear, it is assumed that BSH can target malignant brain tumors by crossing the pathologically permeable blood-brain-barrier (BBB) in the tumor rather than the intact BBB [99]. Based on the above unique characteristics, BSH may not be suitable to treat tumors localized in organs that do not absorb BSH and tumors containing hypoxic/necrotic areas due to its high water solubility. To improve its targeting capacity, BSH is recommended to be conjugated with other drugs.

BPA has been synthesized at industry scale in the Good Manufacturing Practices (GMP) facility for clinical application. For example, in Sunshine Lake Pharma Co. Ltd. in Guangdong, China, the GMP standard process has been built up to produce high-quality BPA, and so far around 70 kg of BPA have been obtained for investigational new drug (IND) applications in China. A few new neutron stations have also been built in China such as BNCT centers in Dongguan General Hospital and Xiamen Hongai Hospital. New generations of the BNCT drugs are highly expected to overcome the drawbacks of BPA and BSH, and accelerate development of BNCT in Asian countries. Indeed, different boron-containing drugs or drug delivery systems have been reported such as boron-containing compounds modified with peptides [100], amino acids [101], carbohydrate analogues [102], porphyrins [103,104], nucleosides [105], liposomes [106] and monoclonal antibodies [107]. The achievements are discussed in the following chapters.

References

1. Wiberg, N. (2001). *Inorganic Chemistry.* Academic Press.
2. https://ciaaw.org/boron.htm.
3. Rizzo, H. F. (1960). Oxidation of Boron at Temperatures between 400 and 1300°C in Air. In: Kohn, J. A., Nye, W. F. and Gaulé, G. K. (Eds.), *Boron Synthesis, Structure, and Properties,* Springer, pp. 175–189.
4. Woods, W. G. (1994). An introduction to boron: history, sources, uses, and chemistry. *Environ. Health. Perspect.* 102(Suppl 7), 5–11.
5. Bellott, B. J., Noh, W., Nuzzo, R. G. and Girolami, G. S. (2009). Nanoenergetic materials: boron nanoparticles from the pyrolysis of decaborane and their functionalization. *Chem. Commun.* 2009(22), 3214–3215.
6. Zhu, Y. and Hosmane, N. S. (2018). Liquid-phase synthesis of boron isocyanates: precursors to boron nanoparticles. *Angew. Chem. Int. Ed.* 57, 14888–14890.
7. Zhu, Y., Prommana, P., Hosmane, N. S., Coghi, P., Uthaipibull, C. and Zhang, Y. (2022). Functionalized boron nanoparticles as potential promising antimalarial agents. *ACS Omega* 7(7), 5864–5869.
8. Rohani, P., Kim, S. and Swihart, M. T. (2016). Boron nanoparticles for room-temperature hydrogen generation from water. *Adv. Energy Mater.* 6, 1502550.
9. Brown, H. C. (1975). *Organic Syntheses via Boranes.* John Wiley & Sons.
10. https://www.nobelprize.org/prizes/chemistry/1976/lipscomb/facts/.
11. Welch, A. J. (2013). The significance and impact of Wade's rules. *Chem. Commun.* 49(35), 3615–3616.
12. Mikhailov, B. M. (1962). The chemistry of diborane. *Russ. Chem. Rev.* 31(4), 207–224.
13. Brown, H. C. and Zweifel, G. (1959). *J. Am. Chem. Soc.* 81(15), 4106–4107.
14. Dunks, G. B., Palmer-Ordonez, K. and Hedaya, E. (1983). Decaborane (14). *Inorg. Synth.* 22, 202–207.
15. Greenwood, N. N. and Earnshaw, A. (1997). *Chemistry of the Elements* (2nd ed.). Butterworth-Heinemann, pp.151–195.
16. Dunks, G. B. and Ordonez, K. P. (1978). A simplified preparation of $B_{10}H_{14}$ from $NaBH_4$. *J. Am. Chem. Soc.* 100(8), 2555–2556.
17. Martin, R. and Buchwald, S. L. (2008). Palladium-catalyzed Suzuki–Miyaura cross-coupling reactions employing dialkylbiaryl phosphine ligands. *Acc. Chem. Res.* 41(11), 1461–1473.
18. Ishiyama, T., Murata, M. and Miyaura, N. (1995). Palladium(0)-catalyzed cross-coupling reaction of alkoxydiboron with haloarenes: a direct procedure for arylboronic esters. *J. Org. Chem.* 60(23), 7508–7510.
19. Shinokubo, H. (2014). Transition metal catalyzed borylation of functional π-systems. *Proc. Jpn. Acad., Ser. B* 90, 1–11.
20. Takagi, J. (2002). Iridium-catalyzed C–H coupling reaction of heteroaromatic compounds with bis(pinacolato)diboron: regioselective synthesis of heteroarylboronates. *Tetrahedron Lett.* 43(32), 5649–5651.

21. Ishiyama, T. (2002). Mild iridium-catalyzed borylation of arenes. high turnover numbers, room temperature reactions, and isolation of a potential intermediate. *J. Am. Chem. Soc.* **124(3)**, 390–391.

22. Ishiyama, T. (2003). Room temperature borylation of arenes and heteroarenes using stoichiometric amounts of pinacolborane catalyzed by iridium complexes in an inert solvent. *Chem. Commun.* **2003(23)**, 2924–2925.

23. Murphy, J. M. (2007). Meta halogenation of 1,3-disubstituted arenes via iridium-catalyzed arene borylation. *J. Am. Chem. Soc.* **129(50)**, 15434–15435.

24. Chen, H., Schlecht, S., Semple, T. C. and Hartwig, J. F. (2000). Thermal, catalytic, regiospecific functionalization of alkanes. *Science* **287(5460)**, 1995–1997.

25. Hartwig, J. F. (2011). Regioselectivity of the borylation of alkanes and arenes. *Chem. Soc. Rev.* **40(4)**, 1992–2002.

26. Miyaura, N. and Suzuki, A. (1979). Stereoselective synthesis of arylated (E)-alkenes by the reaction of alk-1-enylboranes with aryl halides in the presence of palladium catalyst. *J. Chem. Soc. Chem. Commun.* **(19)**, 866–867.

27. Miyaura, N., Yamada, K. and Suzuki, A. (1979). A new stereospecific cross-coupling by the palladium-catalyzed reaction of 1-alkenylboranes with 1-alkenyl or 1-alkynyl halides. *Tetrahedron Lett.* **20(36)**, 3437–3440.

28. Zhu, Y. and Hosmane, N. S. (2015). Nanocatalysis: Recent advances and applications in boron chemistry. *Coord. Chem. Rev.* **293–294**, 357–367.

29. Suzuki, A. (2011). Cross-coupling reactions of organoboranes: an easy way to construct C-C bonds (Nobel Lecture). *Angew. Chem. Int. Ed.* **50**, 6722–6737.

30. Miyaura, N. and Suzuki, A. (1979). Palladium-catalyzed cross-coupling reactions of organoboron compounds. *Chem. Rev.* **95(7)**, 2457–2483.

31. Suzuki, A. (1999). Recent advances in the cross-coupling reactions of organoboron derivatives with organic electrophiles, 1995–1998. *J. Organomet. Chem.* **576 (1–2)**, 147–168.

32. Petasis, N. A. and Akritopoulou, I. (1993). The boronic acid Mannich reaction: A new method for the synthesis of geometrically pure allylamines. *Tetrahedron Lett.* **34(4)**, 583–586.

33. Yu, T., Li, H., Wu, X. and Yang, J. (2012). Progress in Petasis reaction. *Chin. J. Org. Chem.* **32(10)**, 1836–1845.

34. Roush, W. R., Walts, A. E. and Hoong, L. K. (1985). Diastereo- and enantioselective aldehyde addition reactions of 2-allyl-1,3,2-dioxaborolane-4,5-dicarboxylic esters, a useful class of tartrate ester modified allylboronates. *J. Am. Chem. Soc.* **107(26)**, 8186–8190.

35. Roush, W. R., Ando, K., Powers, D. B., Halterman, R. L. and Palkowitz, A. D. (1988). Enantioselective synthesis using diisopropyl tartrate modified (E)- and (Z)-crotylboronates: Reactions with achiral aldehydes. *Tetrahedron Lett.* **29(44)**, 5579–5582.

36. Roush, W. R. and Grover, P. T. (1990). Diisopropyl tartrate (E)-γ-(dimethylphenylsilyl)allylboronate, a chiral allylic alcohol β-carbanion equivalent

for the enantioselective synthesis of 2-butene-1,4-diols from aldehydes. *Tetrahedron Lett.* **31(52)**, 7567–7570.

37. Roush, W. R., Gover, P. T. and Lin, X. (1990). Diisopropyl tartrate modified (E)-γ-[(cyclohexyloxy)dimethylsilyl-allylboronate, a chiral reagent for the stereoselective synthesis of anti 1,2-diols via the formal α-hydroxyallylation of aldehydes. *Tetrahedron Lett.* **31(52)**, 7563–7566.

38. Fernandes, R. A. and Kattanguru, P. (2011). Total synthesis of (*8S,11R,12R*)- and (*8R,11R,12R*)-topsentolide B2 diastereomers and assignment of the absolute configuration. *Tetrahedron: Asymmetry* **22(20–22)**, 1930–1935.

39. Liu, J., Lotesta, S. D. and Sorensen, E. J. (2011). A concise synthesis of the molecular framework of pleuromutilin. *Chem. Commun.* **47**, 1500–1502.

40. Vyvyan, J. R. (1999). An expedient total synthesis of (+/-)-caparratriene. *Tetrahedron Lett.* **40(27)**, 4947–4949.

41. Jin, W., Du, W., Yang, Q., Yu, H., Chen, J. and Yu, Z. (2011). Regio- and stereoselective synthesis of multisubstituted olefins and conjugate dienes by using α-oxo ketene dithioacetals as the building blocks. *Org. Lett.* **13(16)**, 4272–4275.

42. Weires, N. A., Baker, E. L. and Garg, N. K. (2015). Nickel-catalysed Suzuki–Miyaura coupling of amides. *Nat. Chem.* **8(1)**, 75–79.

43. Roesner, S., Blair, D. J. and Aggarwal, V. K. (2015). Enantioselective installation of adjacent tertiary benzylic stereocentres using lithiation–borylation–protodeboronation methodology. Application to the synthesis of bifluranol and fluorohexestrol. *Chem. Sci.* **6**, 3718–3723.

44. Molander, G. A. and Biolatto, B. (2003). Palladium-catalyzed Suzuki–Miyaura cross-coupling reactions of potassium aryl- and heteroaryltrifluoroborates. *J. Org. Chem.* **68(11)**, 4302–4314.

45. Bates, R. (2012). *Roderick Organic Synthesis Using Transition Metals.* John Wiley & Sons.

46. Zhu, Y., Peng, S. C., Emi, A., Shu, Z., Monalisa and Kemp, R. (2007). Supported ultra small palladium on magnetic nanoparticles used as catalysts for Suzuki cross-coupling and Heck reactions. *Adv. Synth. Catal.* **349**, 1917–1922.

47. Chan, D. M. T. (2003). Copper promoted C–N and C–O bond cross-coupling with phenyl and pyridylboronates. *Tetrahedron Lett.* **44(19)**, 3863–3865.

48. Lam, P. Y. S. (2003). Copper-promoted/catalyzed C–N and C–O bond cross-coupling with vinylboronic acid and its utilities. *Tetrahedron Lett.* **44(26)**, 4927–4931.

49. Kolekar, Y. A. and Bhanage, B. M. (2021). Pd-catalyzed oxidative aminocarbonylation of arylboronic acids with unreactive tertiary amines via C-N bond activation. *J. Org. Chem.* **86(20)**, 14208–14035.

50. Yasui, Y., Tsuchida, S., Miyabe, H. and Takemoto, Y. (2007). One-pot amidation of olefins through Pd-catalyzed coupling of alkylboranes and carbamoyl chlorides. *J. Org. Chem.* **72(15)**, 5898–5900.

51. Yin, Z., Wang, Z., Li, W. and Wu, X.-F. (2017). Copper catalyzed carbonylative cross-coupling of arylboronic acids with N-chloroamines for the synthesis of aryl amides. *Eur. J. Org. Chem.* **2017(13)**, 1769–1772.

52. Zhang, J., Hou, Y., Ma, Y. and Szostak, M. (2019). Synthesis of amides by mild palladium-catalyzed aminocarbonylation of arylsilanes with amines enabled by copper(II) fluoride. *J. Org. Chem.* **84(1)**, 338–345.

53. Ren, L., Li, X. and Jiao, N. (2016). Dioxygen-promoted Pd-catalyzed aminocarbonylation of organoboronic acids with amines and CO: A direct approach to tertiary amides. *Org. Lett.* **18(22)**, 5852–5855.

54. Lipscomb, W. N. (1963). *Boron Hydrides.* Benjamin.

55. Lipscomb, W. N. (1966). Framework rearrangement in boranes and carboranes: Cooperative atomic rearrangements are expected in many polyhedron-like electron-deficient molecules and ions. *Science* **153**, 373–378.

56. Grimes, R. N. (2016). *Carboranes* (3rd ed.). Academic Press.

57. Doğan, S. and Akdağ, A. (2020). Studies on synthesis of boron and carborane cage derivatives. *J. Boron* **5(1)**, 1–11.

58. Jemmis, E. D. (1982). Overlap control and stability of polyhedral molecules. Closo-carboranes. *J. Am. Chem. Soc.* **104(25)**, 7017–7020.

59. Zhu, Y. (2022). *Fundamentals and Applications of Boron Chemistry.* Elsevier.

60. Zakharkin, L. I. and Grebennikov, A. V. (1967). *Izv. Akad. Nauk SSSR, Ser. Khim.* 1376–1377.

61. Zakharkin, L. I., Stanko, V. I., Brattsev, V., Yu, A., Chapovskii, A., Klimova, A. I., *et al.* (1964). The synthesis and properties of a new class of organoboron compounds $B_{10}C_2H_{12}$ (baren) and its derivatives. *Dokl. Akad. Nauk SSSR* **155**, 1119–1122.

62. Zakharkin, L. I., Grebennikov, A. V. and Kazantsev, A. V. (1967). Alkylation of carborane Grignard reagents. *Russ. Chem. Bull.* **16**, 1991–1993.

63. Hawthorne, M. F., Young, D. C. and Wegner, P. A. (1965). Carbametallic boron hydride derivatives. I. Apparent analogs of ferrocene and ferricinium ion. *J. Am. Chem. Soc.* **87**, 1818–1819.

64. Zhu, Y. and Hosmane, N. S. (2013). Carborane-based transition metal complexes and their catalytic applications for olefin polymerization: Current and future perspectives. *J. Organomet. Chem.* **747**, 25–29.

65. Stevens, J. C., Timmers, F. J., Wilson, D. R., Schmidt, G. F., Nickias, P. N., Rosen, R. K., *et al.* (1991). *Eur. Pat. Appl.* EP416815A2.

66. Sieckhaus, J. F., Semenuk, N. S., Knowles, T. A. and Schroeder, H. (1969). Icosahedral carboranes. XIII. Halogenation of p-carborane. *Inorg. Chem.* **8**, 2452–2457.

67. Baker, S. J., Tomsho, J. W. and Benkovic, S. J. (2011). Boron-containing inhibitors of synthetases. *Chem. Soc. Rev.* **40(8)**, 4279–4285.

68. Baker, S. J., Ding, C. Z., Akama, T., Zhang, Y.-K., Xia, Y. and Hernandez, V. (2009). Therapeutic potential of boron containing compounds. *Future Med. Chem.* **1**, 1275–1288.

69. Adams, J., Behnke, M., Chen, S. W., Cruickshank, A. A., Dick, L. R., Grenier, L., et al. (1998). Potent, selective inhibitors of the proteasome: Dipeptidyl boronic acids. *Bioorg. Med. Chem. Lett.* **8**, 333–338.

70. Adamczyk-Woźniak, A., Borys, K. M. and Sporzyński, A. (2015). Recent developments in the chemistry and biological applications of benzoxaboroles. *Chem. Rev.* **115**, 5224–5247.

71. https://www.businesswire.com/news/home/20140708005679/en/FDA-Approves-Anacor-Pharmaceuticals%E2%80%99-KERYDIN%E2%84%A2-Tavaborole-Topical-Solution-5-for-the-Treatment-of-Onychomycosis-of-the-Toenails.

72. Shirley, M. (2016). Ixazomib: first global approval. *Drugs* **76**, 405–411.

73. Hoy, S. M. (2017). Crisaborole ointment 2%: a review in mild to moderate atopic dermatitis. *Am. J. Clin. Dermatol.* **18**, 837–843.

74. https://www.accessdata.fda.gov/drugsatfda_docs/label/2017/209776lbl.pdf.

75. *Scifinder*, version 2019; Chemical Abstracts Service: Columbus, OH, 2019; RN 58-08-2 (accessed March, 2019).

76. Coghi, P. S., Zhu, Y., Xie, H., Hosmane, N. S. and Zhang, Y. (2021). Organoboron compounds: Effective antibacterial and antiparastic agents. *Molecules* **26**, 3309.

77. Sponseller, J. K., Griffiths, J. K. and Tzipori, S. (2014). The evolution of respiratory Cryptosporidiosis: evidence for transmission by inhalation. *Clin. Microbiol. Rev.* **27**(3), 575–586.

78. https://www.who.int/water_sanitation_health/gdwqrevision/cryptodraft2.pdf.

79. Dubey, J. P. (2014). Chapter 1 — The History and Life Cycle of Toxoplasma gondii. In: Weiss, L. M. (Ed.), *Toxoplasma Gondii* (2nd ed.), Academic Press, pp. 1–17.

80. Lv, P.-C. and Zhu, H.-L. (2012). Aminoacyl-tRNA synthetase inhibitors as potent antibacterials. *Curr. Med. Chem.* **19**, 3550–3563.

81. Palencia, A., Liu, R. J., Lukarska, M., Gut, J., Bougdour, A., Touquet, B., et al. (2016). Cryptosporidium and Toxoplasma parasites are inhibited by a benzoxaborole targeting leucyl-tRNA synthetase. *Antimicrob. Agents Chemother.* **60**(10), 5817–5827.

82. Barth, R. F., Mi, P. and Yang, W. (2018). Boron delivery agents for neutron capture therapy of cancer. *Cancer Commun.* **38**(1), 35.

83. Dymova, M. A., Taskaev, S. Y., Richter, V. A. and Kuligina, E. V. (2020). Boron neutron capture therapy: Current status and future perspectives. *Cancer Commun.* **40**(9), 406–421.

84. Takahara, K., Miyatake, S.-I., Azuma, H. and Shiroki, R. (2022). Boron neutron capture therapy for urological cancers. *Int. J. Urology* **29**, 610–616.

85. Monti, H. A. (2022). Importance of radiobiological studies for the advancement of boron neutron capture therapy (BNCT). *Expert. Rev. Mol. Med.* **24**, e14.

86. Jalilian, A. R., Shahi, A., Swainson, I. P., Nakamura, H., Venkatesh, M. and Osso, J. A. (2022). Potential theranostic boron neutron capture therapy agents as multimodal radiopharmaceuticals. *Cancer Biother. Radiopharm.* **37**, 342–354.

87. Hu, K., Yang, Z., Zhang, L., Xie, L., Wang, L., Xu, H., *et al.* (2020). Boron agents for neutron capture therapy. *Coord. Chem. Rev.* **405**, 213139.
88. Pitto-Barry, A. (2021). Polymers and boron neutron capture therapy (BNCT): a potent combination. *Poly. Chem.* **12**, 2035–2044.
89. Seneviratne, D., Advani, P., Trifiletti, D. M., Chumsri, S., Beltran, C. J., Bush, A. F. and Vallow, L. A. (2022). Exploring the biological and physical basis of boron neutron capture therapy (BNCT) as a promising treatment frontier in breast cancer. *Cancers (Basel)* **14(12)**, 3009.
90. Hosmane, N. S., Maguire, J. A., Zhu, Y. and Takagaki, M. (Eds.) (2012). *Boron and Gadolinium Neutron Capture Therapy for Cancer Treatment.* World Scientific.
91. Farr, L. E., Sweet, W. H., Robertson, J. S., Foster, C. G., Locksley, H. B., Sutherland, D. L., *et al.* (1954). Neutron capture therapy with boron in the treatment of glioblastoma multiforme. *Am. J. Roentgenol. Radium. Ther. Nucl. Med.* **71**, 279–293.
92. Soloway, A. H., Hatanaka, H. and Davis, M. A. (1967). Penetration of brain and brain tumor. VII. Tumor-binding sulfhydryl boron compounds. *J. Med. Chem.* **10**, 714–717.
93. Hatanaka, H. (1990). Clinical Results of Boron Neutron Capture Therapy. In: Harling, O. K., Bernard, J. A. and Zamenhof, R. G. (Eds.), *Neutron Beam Design, Development, and Performance for Neutron Capture Therapy*, Springer, pp. 15–21.
94. Snyder, H. R., Reedy, A. J. and Lennarz, W. J. (1958). Synthesis of aromatic boronic acids. Aldehydo boronic acids and a boronic acid analog of Tyrosine1. *J. Am. Chem. Soc.* **80**, 835–838.
95. Wang, L. W., Chen, Y. W., Ho, C. Y., Hsueh Liu, Y. W., Chou, F. I., Liu, Y. H., *et al.* (2016). Fractionated boron neutron capture therapy in locally recurrent head and neck cancer: a prospective phase I/II trial. *Int. J. Radiat. Oncol. Biol. Phys.* **95**, 396–403.
96. Coderre, J. A., Button, T. M., Micca, P. L., Fisher, C. D., Nawrocky, M. M. and Liu, H. B. (1994). Neutron capture therapy of the 9l rat gliosarcoma using the P-boronophenylalanine-fructose complex. *Int. J. Radiat. Oncol. Biol. Phys.* **30(3)**, 643–652.
97. Wongthai, P., Hagiwara, K., Miyoshi, Y., Wiriyasermkul, P., Wei, L., Ohgaki, R., *et al.* (2015). Boronophenylalanine, a boron delivery agent for boron neutron capture therapy, is transported by $ATB^{0,}+$, LAT1 and LAT2. *Cancer Sci.* **106(3)**, 279–286.
98. Puris, E., Gynther, M., Auriola, S. and Huttunen, K. M. (2020). L-type amino acid transporter 1 as a target for drug delivery. *Pharm. Res.* **37(5)**, 88.
99. Wittig, A., Stecher-Rasmussen, F., Hilger, R. A., Rassow, J., Mauri, P. and Sauerwein, W. (2011). Sodium mercaptoundecahydro-closo-dodecaborate (BSH), a boron carrier that merits more attention. *Appl. Radiat. Isot.* **69(12)**, 1760–1764.

100. Hoppenz, P., Els-Heindl, S., Kellert, M., Kuhnert, R., Saretz, S., Lerchen, H.-G., et al. (2020). A selective carborane-functionalized gastrin-releasing peptide receptor agonist as boron delivery agent for boron neutron capture therapy. J. Org. Chem. **85**, 1446–1457.

101. Gruzdev, D. A., Levit, G. L., Krasnov, V. P. and Charushin, V. N. (2021). Carborane-containing amino acids and peptides: Synthesis, properties and applications. Coord. Chem. Rev. **433**, 213753.

102. Tsurubuchi, T., Shirakawa, M., Kurosawa, W., Matsumoto, K., Ubagai, R., Umishio, H., et al. (2020). Evaluation of a novel boron-containing α-d-mannopyranoside for BNCT. Cells **9**, 1277.

103. Shi, Y., Li, J., Zhang, Z., Duan, D., Zhang, Z., Liu, H., et al. (2018). Tracing boron with fluorescence and positron emission tomography imaging of boronated porphyrin nanocomplex for imaging-guided boron neutron capture therapy. ACS Appl. Mater. Interfaces **10**, 43387–43395.

104. Bhupathiraju, N. V. S. D. K. and Vicente, M. G. H. (2013). Synthesis and cellular studies of polyamine conjugates of a mercaptomethyl–carboranylporphyrin. Bioorg. Med. Chem. **21**, 485–495.

105. Uram, Ł., Nizioł, J., Maj, P., Sobich, J., Rode, W. and Ruman, T. (2017). N(4)-[B-(4,4,5,5-tetramethyl-1,3,2-dioxaborolan)methyl]-2′-deoxycytidine as a potential boron delivery agent with respect to glioblastoma. Biomed. Pharmacother. **95**, 749–755.

106. Luderer, M. J., Muz, B., Alhallak, K., Sun, J., Wasden, K., Guenthner, N., et al. (2019). Thermal sensitive liposomes improve delivery of boronated agents for boron neutron capture therapy. Pharm. Res. **36(10)**, 144.

107. Wu, G., Barth, R. F., Yang, W., Chatterjee, M., Tjarks, W., Ciesielski, M. J. and Fenstermaker, R. A. (2004). Site-specific conjugation of boron-containing dendrimers to anti-EGF receptor monoclonal antibody cetuximab (IMC-C225) and its evaluation as a potential delivery agent for neutron capture therapy. Bioconjugate Chem. **15**, 185–194.

https://doi.org/10.1142/9789811268038_0002

Chapter 2

Boron Neutron Capture Therapy in Clinical Trials

Fayaz Ali,[1] Yinghuai Zhu[2,*]

[1] *Department of Chemistry, Gomal University Sub-Campus Tank, Pakistan*
[2] *Sunshine Lake Pharma Co. Ltd., China*

Abstract

Boron Neutron Capture Therapy (BNCT) is one of the most promising treatments among NCTs due to its long-term clinical application and unequivocal success in clinical trials. Nevertheless, current clinically used boronophenylalanine suffers from large uptake dose and low blood-to-tumor selectivity, and that initiated an overwhelming screening of next-generation BNCT drugs. Various boron agents, such as small molecules and macro/nano-vehicles, have been explored to greater success. In this chapter, different types of agents are rationally analyzed and compared, and the feasible targets are shared to present a perspective for the future of BNCT in cancer treatment.

Keywords: Boron neutron capture therapy, boron drug, antitumor treatment, clinical application, drug delivery.

2.1 BNCT in Cancer Therapy

2.1.1 *Introduction*

The actual advancement in medicinal chemistry of boron started from the use of boron neutron capture therapy (BNCT) for cancer [1,2]. The

---

* Corresponding author.

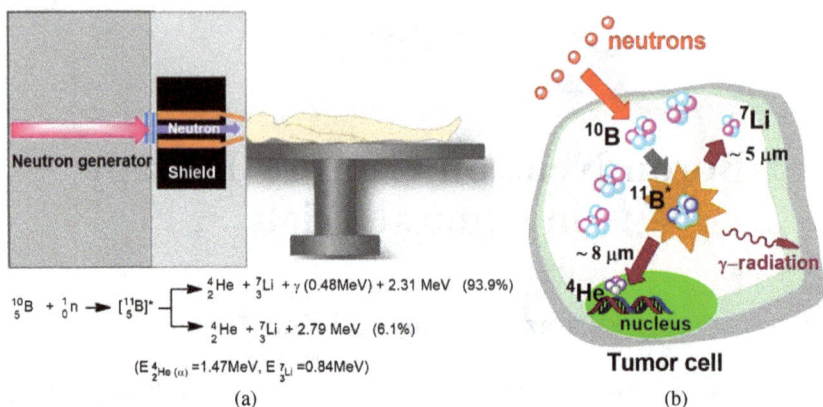

$$\overset{10}{_{5}}B + \overset{1}{_{0}}n \longrightarrow [\overset{11}{_{5}}B]^* \overset{\nearrow}{\searrow} \quad \begin{array}{l} \overset{4}{_{2}}He + \overset{7}{_{3}}Li + \gamma\,(0.48\text{MeV}) + 2.31\text{ MeV} \quad (93.9\%) \\[4pt] \overset{4}{_{2}}He + \overset{7}{_{3}}Li + 2.79\text{ MeV} \quad (6.1\%) \end{array}$$

$$(E_{\overset{4}{_{2}}He\,(\alpha)} = 1.47\text{MeV}, \; E_{\overset{7}{_{3}}Li} = 0.84\text{MeV})$$

(a)

(b)

Figure 2.1 (a) Schematic illustration of the BNCT system. (b) Schematic diagram of the cell-killing mechanism of BNCT.

clinical treatment of cancers with the help of BNCT is linked to the development in nuclear research technology and the availability of suitable neutron sources. A schematic diagram of a BNCT device is shown in Figure 2.1(a). BNCT is based on the nuclear capture and fission reactions that occur when the stable isotope boron-10 (^{10}B) is irradiated with either low-energy (0.025 eV) thermal neutrons, or with epithermal neutrons (10,000 eV) for clinical studies, which become thermalized as they penetrate tissues. During this process, high-linear energy transfer α particles (^{4}He) and recoiling lithium-7 (^{7}Li) nuclei are produced as shown in Figure 2.1(b). For successful delivery, at least ~20 µg/g of ^{10}B per weight of tumor must be selectively delivered to the tumor cells (~10^9 atoms/cell), and enough neutrons must be absorbed by them to sustain a lethal ^{10}B(n, α)^{7}Li capture reaction [1]. Due to very short pathlengths (5–9 µm) of α particles, their destructive effects are limited to boron-containing cells. In principle, α particles can spare normal cells and selectively destroy tumor cells. Interest of BNCT in clinical use is focused primarily on patients with recurrent tumors of high-grade gliomas [2–5] and of the head and neck region [6–13], whom conventional therapies have failed. In addition, BNCT is applied on a smaller number of patients with lung cancer and cutaneous [14–17] or extra-cutaneous [18] melanomas.

A major area of inorganic-organic metallic chemistry has been developed from the study of electron-deficient boron clusters, which now considerably overlay with medicinal and organic chemistry. The mission of BNCT was facilitated in the 1960s by the discovery of new polyhedral boron compounds which contain clusters of boron instead of a single boron atom per molecule [4–7]. These polyhedral boranes emerged as new boron carrier candidates for BNCT. Among the new compounds of low molecular weight produced for BNCT were carbo-rane-containing carbohydrates, amino acids, nucleosides, nucleic acids and bases, lipids, DNA groove binders, and porphyrins [4–7]. Recently, a new generation of radiosensitizers was described for BNCT which includes biopolymers containing one or more carbonyl deposits. This class of boron contains nucleic acids (DNA-oligonucleotides), carbonyl oligophosphates, and carbonyl peptides and proteins [6,8,9].

Basic knowledge about pharmacokinetics and toxicity of boron compounds has been achieved by broad studies on boron carriers for BNCT, which proved useful for the development of boron compounds for other biological applications. For instance, new biological activities of boron cage molecules and their complexes have been revealed, including anti-HIV activity, anti-rheumatoid arthritis activity, drug delivery and imaging for diagnosis and treatment of cancer, and probing protein-biomolecule interactions [10–13].

These and other outcomes clearly exhibit that boron-containing compounds have great unexplored potential in medical applications and bioorganic chemistry. It's not essential that for every drug discovery problem, boron is to be the solution; however, it will be a good addition to the toolbox of medicinal chemistry. About three decades ago, fluorine had the same status in medicinal chemistry as boron currently, yet now compounds of fluorine are synthesized on a routine basis in pharmaceutical research, and occupy a considerable role in the pharmaceutical market. Various reviews and books have been recently published showing the advances in boron chemistry and its applications [9,13–26], but here we are hoping to spotlight the immense applications of boron chemistry by focusing on the neutron capture therapy drugs for cancer treatment.

2.1.2 Brain Tumor

BNCT for brain tumor was performed for the first time in the U.S. in the 1950s at Brookhaven National Laboratory [27,28]. However, the patients' median survival after BNCT was only 87 days. In the 1990s, epithermal beams became available for BNCT in the U.S., Japan, Germany, Czech Republic, Sweden, Finland and Taiwan. As a result, the therapeutic possibilities and biological effects of BNCT improved. It was reported that when treating 167 cases of high-grade meningiomas and malignant brain tumors using BNCT with boronophenylalanine (BPA), the median survival time for recurrent glioblastoma was 10.8 months, while using BNCT with BPA and sodium borocaptate (BSH) was 23.5 months with an X-ray boost and 15.6 months without an X-ray boost [29].

Recently, BNCT was applied on 34 patients with life-threatening, end-stage brain tumors as reported by Chen *et al.* [30]. No severe adverse events were observed (grade $\geq$ 3). The objective response and disease control rates were 50.0% and 85.3%, respectively. The mean overall survival (OS), cancer-specific survival, and relapse-free survival times were 7.25, 7.80, and 4.18 months, respectively.

A cyclotron-based accelerator neutron source was constructed by Sumitomo Heavy Industries and approved by the Ministry of Health, Labor and Welfare of Japan in March 2020 [31]. The safety and efficacy of such accelerator-based BNCT was assessed in 27 patients with recurrent glioblastoma by Kawabata *et al.* [32]. The 1-year survival rate and median OS were 79.2% and 18.9 months, respectively.

Recently, a boron delivery system that involves the cerebrospinal fluid (CSF) was developed to improve the therapeutic efficacy of BNCT, in contrast to the conventional method which involves intravenous (IV) administration [33]. The study used BPA and monitored the uptake rate of boron by the brain cells as well as the time-concentration profile of boron in the CSF of normal rats. Comparable brain cell uptake levels were achieved with CSF-based and IV administration methods; however, lower BPA doses were involved in the former method. These findings suggest that the economic and physical burdens may be reduced by using the CSF method for brain tumor patients.

2.1.3 Head and Neck Cancer

Inoperable, locally advanced head and neck cancer patients were treated with BNCT in clinical phase I/II trial between December 2003 and September 2008 in Finland as reported by Kankaanranta et al. [34]. The response rate was 76% and the median progression-free survival time was 7.5 months, with a 2-year OS. In another study Koivunoro et al. reported 79 patients of locally recurrent head and neck inoperable squamous cell carcinoma treated with BPA-mediated BNCT in Finland between February 2003 and January 2012. 68% of these patients showed some recovery, with a 36% complete response rate. The 2-year locoregional progression-free survival rate was 38%, and the OS rate was 21% [35].

2.1.4 Hepatocellular Carcinoma

The first case of a patient treated for multiple hepatocellular carcinomas was in Japan, reported by Suzuki et al. [36]. Because of compromised liver function, the multiple tumors in the left liver lobe with hepatic arterial chemoembolization and in the right liver lobe were treated with BNCT. For 1 month, the tumors treated with BNCT remained stable in size. Unfortunately, due to liver dysfunction caused by progression of hepatocellular carcinoma, the patient died 10 months after BNCT.

The first case of multiple hepatocellular carcinomas in the left liver lobe treated with BNCT involving selective intra-arterial infusion of a BSH-containing water-in-oil-in-water emulsion was reported by Yangie et al. [37]. The tumorous region size remained stable for 3 months; however, due to tumor progression he died after 7 months of BNCT.

2.1.5 Malignant Mesothelioma and Lung Cancer

BNCT has been shown to be a possible lung cancer treatment [38–40]. BNCT therapeutic effect was demonstrated on lung metastases from colon carcinoma and clear cell sarcoma in animal models, with no toxicity in normal tissues [40,41]. The feasibility of BPA-F in BNCT for inoperable malignant pleural mesothelioma was reported by Suzuki et al. [42–44]. BNCT was applied on two patients, one with a malignant short spindle cell tumor and one with malignant pleural mesothelioma [42]. The size of the tumor remained stable for 3–6 months with no late toxicities and no grade 3 or higher acute. BPA-BNCT with nicotinamide (a hypoxia-releasing agent) or bevacizumab was found to enhance the reduction in lung metastases [45]. In another study, BPA-BNCT in combination with both tirapazamine and mild temperature hyperthermia as well as nicotinamide reduced the number of lung metastases, whereas BSH-BNCT combined with a hypoxic cytotoxin, tirapazamine, with or without mild temperature hyperthermia (that improves tumor oxygenation) improved local tumor control [46]. Furthermore, BNCT has also been applied for treating shallow lung tumor as reported by Farias *et al.* [47]. It was postulated that control of the chronic hypoxia-rich Q cell population in the primary solid tumor has the potential to impact the control of local tumors as a whole and that control of the acute hypoxia-rich total tumor cell population in the primary solid tumor has the potential to impact the control of lung metastases [45].

2.1.6 Skin Melanoma

BNCT in melanoma treatments was reported to be useful and sensitive [48], in contrast to conventional radiotherapy which is characterized by highly non-uniform dose distributions in the skin. In Argentina, seven patients (six females and one male) of multiple subcutaneous skin metastases of melanoma with an average age of 64 years (51–74) were treated between October 2003 and June 2007 [49]. All patients received an infusion containing ~14 g/m^2 of BPA followed by a mixed thermal-epithermal neutron beam. 69.3% overall response rate was recorded, with 3 out of 10 evaluable areas showing ulceration (30% toxicity grade 3), which suggests that the toxicity was acceptable. Recently, [10]B-enriched BPA-fructose complex infusion was studied on three skin melanomas of BNCT patients [50]. Tumor/blood (T/B) and skin/blood (S/B) ratios were measured to determine [10]B concentration in tumor, blood and skin. S/B ratio for the patients was in the range 0.81–1.99 and T/B was in the range 1.48–3.82. The T/B ratio of nodular metastasis melanoma was confirmed to be higher than superficial spreading melanoma. And ^{10}B concentration in skin was greater than blood, which is useful to evade overdose in normal skin. Preclinical magnetic resonance imaging (MRI)-guided BNCT was performed on skin melanomas, head and neck recurrent and primary cancers, and highly malignant brain tumors [51]. More recently, valproic acid (VPA) (a promising sensitizer for cancer therapies) was used in concurrence with BNCT to enhance the effect of destroying melanoma cells [52]. The results showed that combining action of VPA and BNCT could considerably constrain the growth of melanoma cells.

2.2 Importance of the Boron Drug in BNCT

The unavailability of tumor-specific BNCT drugs with sufficient tumor uptake is one of the major limitations in BNCT. An ideal boron-based compound must satisfy a few conditions to be used in BNCT, such as high tumor/tissue and tumor/blood concentration ratios (> 2.5:1), low toxicity in the living system, tumor concentrations of 20–35 μg ^{10}B/g tumor, and speedy clearance from healthy tissue and blood. However, its persistence is necessary in the tumor for some hours while being irradiated with neutrons [53].

Over time, to improve low systemic toxicity with targeting tumor cells, three generations of boron compounds have been evolved. Boric acid and its derivatives, which were used in clinical trials during the 1950s–1960s, are considered as first generation. These compounds showed poor tumor retention time, low selectivity and imperfect tumor/brain ratios. BPA and BSH are considered as second-generation compounds which remained longer in tumors, displayed considerably lower toxicity, and achieved the desirable tumor/brain and tumor/blood ratios. These are still used in clinical trials. For instance, sorbitol-BPA injectable solution approved in Japan in May 2020 (Steboronine) is based on advances in drug formulations on this generation of compounds. Development of boron clusters connected through a hydrolytically stable linkage with a tumor-targeting component or moiety is considered as the third-generation compounds. Third-generation agents include one or more polyhedral anions of borane or carboranes, which will be discussed further in this chapter [54,55].

2.3 New Boron Agents Developed for BNCT

To date, two boron compounds, BPA and BSH, have been successfully applied in BNCT clinical trials [56]. Structures of BPA and BSH are shown in Figure 2.2. BPA is an amino acid derivative actively incorporated into tumor cells by the L-type amino acid transporter 1. On the other hand, BSH is a water-soluble diffusive drug, principally used for malignant glioma. It does not cross the blood brain barrier (BBB) into normal brain, but accumulates in malignant brain tumors [57]. However, accumulation of BSH in tumor cells is low as BSH has poor membrane permeability [57,58].

Despite their clinical use, both compounds exhibit several limitations. In this sense, new boron delivery agents are under development, such as liposomes [59], monoclonal antibodies [60], nanoparticles [61,62], carrier proteins conjugated with boron compounds [63], boron cluster agents [64] and bimodal drugs (with anti-tumoral and BNCT effects) such as metallocarboranes [65,66]. To date, in clinical trials boron concentration in tumor cells has been estimated using empirical data models depending on tumor/normal tissue, tumor/ blood and normal tissue/blood concentration ratios. However, in tumors the uptake and concentration of boron varies among patients.

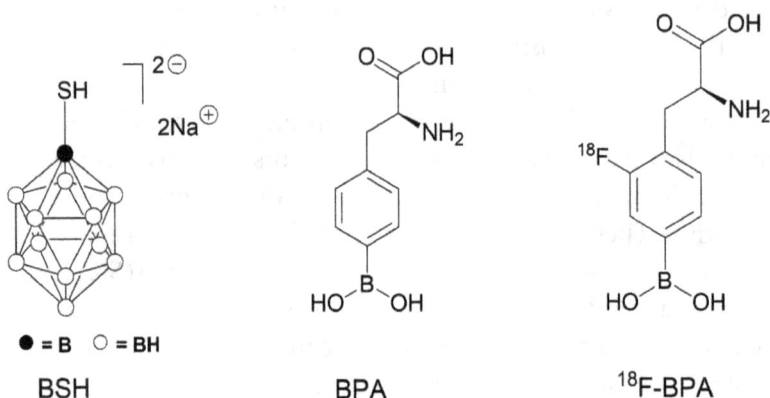

Figure 2.2 Structures of BSH, BPA and ^{18}F-BPA.

Recently, high-precision treatment and indications were developed using high-resolution imaging to monitor and determine the boron uptake in real time for each patient and each tumor [67–69]. The o-[^{18}F]-fluoro-L-p-boronophenylalanine ([^{18}F]-L-FBPA), an ^{18}F-labelled radiopharmaceutical analogue of L-BPA, has been used as a positron emission tomography (PET) probe (Figure 2.2) [70]. However, this compound showed limitations [71]. Therefore, an enormous struggle is dedicated to the development of new theranostic compounds of BNCT; for example, metal nanoparticle hybrids coated with m-carboranylphosphinate [61], iron–boron (Fe–B) nanoparticles [62], and many more. Halogenated carborane derivatives are one of the examples that have been shown to provide nuclear imaging by PET-CT (positron emission tomography-computed tomography, ^{124}I, a positron emitter) and SPECT (single photon emission computed tomography, ^{125}I, a gamma emitter) [4,72]. However, to approve an ideal and promising boron carrier will require years of studies and high cost to be fit for treatment [40]. Moreover, the therapeutic efficacy may be enhanced only by deeper understanding of the radiobiological mechanisms induced by BNCT, which may serve to modulate signaling pathways [73,74].

Efforts have been made towards the development of efficient ^{10}B delivery vehicles to target tumor vasculature [75,76]. For example, flavone acetic acid (FAA) combined with BSH were explored as a selective inhibitor of tumor blood flow in a squamous cell carcinoma (SCC) model [77]. FAA inhibited the clearance of BSH from the tumor but had little or no effect in normal tissue. ZD6126 (N-acetylcochinol-O-phosphate) was reported as another vascular targeting agent, which in combination with BNCT enhanced the sensitivity of the quiescent (Q) tumor cells compared with the total tumor cells in an SCC model in mice [78]. More recently, annexin A1-targeting IFLLWQR (IF7)-conjugated ^{10}BPA or ^{10}BSH in bladder tumor-bearing mice was studied by Yoneyama et $al.$ [79], and demonstrated an enhancement in the therapeutic efficacy versus BPA and BSH alone. Some of the available boron agents and their methods for analysis and imaging of the typical applications in BNCT are shown in Table 2.1.

Table 2.1 Available boron agents and methods for analysis and imaging of the typical applications in BNCT.

Boron Agent	Sample Form and Preparation Method	Analytical Method*	Model	Ref.
BSH	biological tissue in pure Teflon tubes	PGRA	healthy rabbits' brain tissue	[80]
	tissue after digestion	DCP-AES	melanoma-bearing mice	[81]
	freeze-dried sections	EELS	human melanoma cells	[82]
	urine and plasma samples	FI/ESI-MS/MS	patients with a tumor squamous cell	[83]
	rats' liver tissue	¹⁰B-NMR	mice with implanted M2R melanoma	[84]
BPA	biological tissue	ICP-MS	cancerous lesions and tumor-free tissue of the patient's liver	[85]
	freeze-dried cell samples	nano-SIMS	primary cell cultures from human patients exhibiting glioblastoma multiform	[86]
	localized node-negative scalp-angiosarcoma	accelerator-based BNCT	Scalp-angiosarcoma of the two patients with largest diameter of the tumor ≤ 15 cm	[87]
¹⁰BPA		¹⁸F-BPA PET	20 patients with squamous cell carcinoma of the head and neck and 8 patients with malignant melanoma	[88]
BSH, BPA	tumor cell suspensions	PGRA	rodent SCC VII carcinoma tumor-bearing mice	[78]
	tissue digested by nitric acid solution	ICP-AES	C6 glioma-bearing rats	[89]
	tissue embedded in epoxy resin	QNCR	C6 glioma-bearing rats	[90]
	freezing sample	laser-SIMS	nude mice with murine sarcoma	[91]
BSSB	sample with laser beam	SIRIMP & LARIMP	tumor-bearing rats	[92]
	rats' liver tissue	¹¹B-NMR	healthy rats' liver tissue	[93]
cis-ABCPC	cryosections	SIMS	B16 mouse model and F98 rat glioma model	[94]
carborane	rats' liver tissue	MRI	AH109A tumor-bearing rats	[95]

*BPA = L-boronophenylalanine, BSH = mercaptoundeca-hydrododecaborate-¹⁰BSH, BSSB = BSH disulfide, cis-ABCPC = cis-1-amino-3-borono-cyclopentanecarboxylic acid, PGRA = prompt β-ray analysis, DCP-AES = direct-current plasma atomic emission spectroscopy, EELS = electron energy loss spectroscopy, ICP-AES = inductively coupled plasma atomic emission spectrometry, QNCR = quantitative neutron capture radiography, SIMS = secondary ion mass spectrometry, SIRIMP = sputter-initiated resonance ionization microprobe, LARIMP = laser atomization resonance ionization microprobe, PET = positron emission tomography, NMR = nuclear magnetic resonance, MRI = magnetic resonance imaging.

Boron nitride has emerged as an advanced and innovative material which can be used for cancer treatment in BNCT [96]. For instance, Sing et al. [97] reported highly water-dispersible boron nitride nanostructures with ultra-high disperse ability and structural deformation that were very much useful for BNCT. In addition, it is reported that controlled boron release and crystallinity of hollow boron nitride spheres increase prostate cancer cell apoptosis and decrease cell viability [98]. Moreover, hexagonal boron nitride (h-BN, similar to graphite "white graphene") is one of the most exceptional layered nanomaterials. In the h-BN structure, the only difference from graphite is the replacement of carbon atoms by boron and nitrogen. This, however, results in an increased band gap which bestows the material with semi-conductive properties which permits their use in biosensors and contrast agents [99,100]. Emanet et al. [101] recently examined the h-BN therapeutic efficiency against prostate cancer. It was reported that h-BN nanomaterials were suitable for cellular internalization with an average size of 50 nm. Results indicate a serious suppressive effect on cancer cells, which was directly proportional to the h-BN concentration.

Other than therapeutic efficiency, the imaging capability of the drug construct is also an important point of consideration. Gadolinium-157 (^{157}Gd) is reported as a potential element for NCT, because of its better image contrast in T1-weighted MRI and toxic effects on tumor cells [102]. Novel boron-containing nanoparticles were developed by scientists using mesoporous silica or gold nanoparticles combined with Gd [103–105]. Recently, to realize multiple functions in one molecule, a new structure of gadolinium-boron capture agent with double effect was developed by grafting ^{10}BSH with Gd [3]. In addition, iron-boron (Fe-B) nanoparticles were generated by Torresan et al. and MRI performed by exploiting the magnetic response of the nanoparticles [62]. By comparing different techniques and studies it is found that FBPA-PET is a useful and reliable imaging tool for BNCT treatment [106]. To simultaneously achieve ^{18}FBPA-PET imaging function and selective delivery of boron to prostate cancer, Meher and his research team designed polymer nanoparticles loaded with carborane and tethered to the radiometal chelator deferoxamine boron [107]. Several research

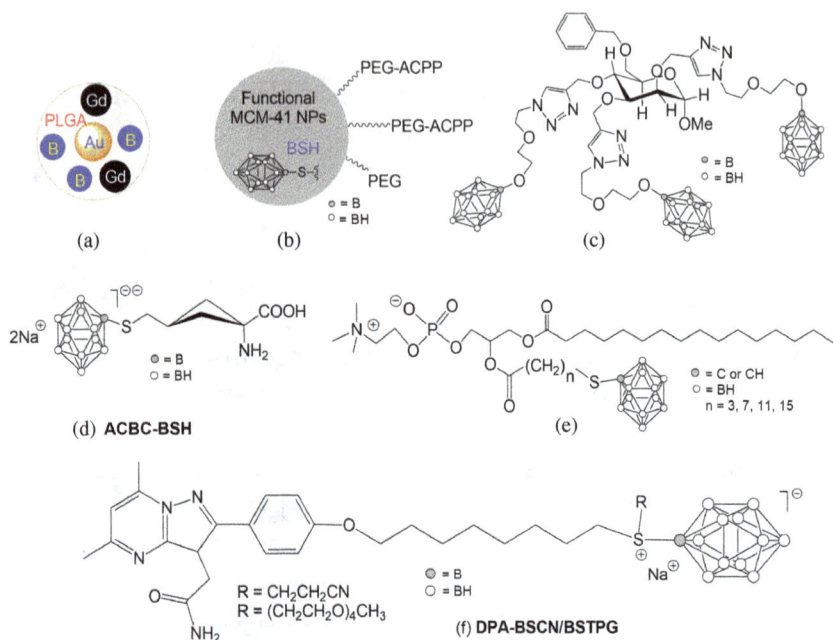

Figure 2.3 (a) The structure of self-synthesized thiol B cage (BC-PLGA-SH)-functionalized Au nanoparticles. (b) Functional mesoporous silica MCM-41 nanoparticles (NPs) conjugated with BSH, PEG, and ACPP. (c) Molecular structure of [10]B-MMT1242. (d) Molecular structure of a BSH derivative ACBC-BSH. (e) Boronated phospholipid. (f) The molecular structure of BSH conjugated with translocator protein ligand.

groups have further continued investigations on optimizing the delivery of BPA and boron clusters by monitoring the distribution of boron using fluorophores [108,109]. Some of the recently reported boron-based complexes are presented in Figure 2.3.

Compound C (Figure 2.3) was synthesized from 1,3,5-triazine-galactopyranoglycinate and carboxylic acids conjugated with nucleophilic side chains [108]. It was claimed that C could effectively accumulate in tumor cells. It showed a high boron uptake, low toxicity and good tumor-to-normal tissue accumulation ratio [108]. Compound

D was reported as a tumor-selective synthetic amino acid [110]. Liu *et al.* reported a carboranylphosphatidycholine-based boronated phospholipid (E) as a boron delivery agent with high biocompatibility, stability and tumor accumulation [111]. The BSH species were also conjugated with translocator protein ligand to improve bio-selectivity (F) [112]. These compounds provide a significant quantity of boron to cancer cells with high water solubility and tumor cell-killing effects for BNCT.

Approaches have also been taken to couple BNCT to other therapies, with encouraging results. For instance, BNCT was combined with thalidomide treatment in the hamster cheek pouch oral cancer model, achieving 100% tumor response with 87% complete tumor remission [113]. Furthermore, electroporation associated with the administration of GB-10 (decahydrodecaborate) was studied for boron delivery and distribution in a hamster model of oral cancer [114]. In another study, it was shown that BNCT and electroporation could be clinically useful [57]. The efficiency of BNCT for oral SCC was enhanced by sonoporation in nude mice by modulating the microlocalization of BPA and BSH in tumors and increasing their intracellular levels [115]. In an orthotopic human oral SCC animal model, a combination of BNCT with low dose gamma irradiation increased BPA accumulation in tumors, thus augmenting BNCT efficacy and extending the overall survival rate [116].

In addition, the possibility of radiosensitisers in combination with particle therapies and BNCT has been explored [117,118]. For example, a histone deacetylase inhibitor, sodium butyrate, increased tumor boron concentration and acted as a radiosensitiser of BPA-BNCT for poorly differentiated thyroid carcinoma [119]. Photosensitisers were also surveyed to combine BNCT and photodynamic therapy [120]. The combined effect of rapamycin and BPA-BNCT on the radiosensitivity of human oral cancer cells was examined by Tatebe *et al.* [121]. Rapamycin inhibits the PI3K/AKT/mTOR pathway, inducing tumor growth inhibition.

Another strategy which needs to be considered is a combination of BNCT and immunotherapy. When a primary tumor is exposed to ionizing radiation, it can induce immunogenic cell death that may in turn activate cytotoxic immune response against the primary tumor and its metastasis. An "out of field" inhibitory effect on tumor growth is called abscopal effect. The abscopal effect of BPA-BNCT was first described by Trivillin *et al.* [122] in an ectopic model of colon cancer in BDIX rats. He further demonstrated that a combination of BNCT with Bacillus Calmette–Guerin (BCG) in the same model could enhance the immune response [123]. The combination of BNCT and BCG might act as an 'anti-tumor vaccine' where BCG would promote antigen presentation in an inflammatory microenvironment and BNCT would trigger the process of tumor antigen generation.

Carboranes are regarded as exceptional boron-containing agents for BNCT because they can potentially deliver high concentrations of boron to tumor sites. Recently, the metallacarborane cobalt bis(dicarbollide), or COSAN, has been investigated for its application in nuclear imaging, whereby in between two dicarbollide moieties a transition metal atom such as Co, Fe or Cr is sandwiched. For potential application in BNCT, studying the biodistribution patterns of radiolabeled carboranes will assist in the elucidation of therapeutic efficacy. For instance, *in vivo* biodistribution studies in mice with dissection and gamma counting using multimodal imaging that combines PET with computed tomography (CT), known as PET-CT, were carried out with the [124]I-labelled COSAN derivative [124–127]. Similarly, a novel radioiodinated bifunctional COSAN derivative that has an iodine atom and a PEG chain has been developed in which both [124]I and ^{125}I isotopes were used for radiolabeling [126].

In the medicinal community, BNCT has been used for a long time; however, clinical investigation of BNCT agents are very much limited. The causes include limited geographical distribution of research reactors; absence of new and high-specificity BNCT agents; limited number of malignancies that can be practically treated with BNCT; dosimetry aspects of tumor geometry and neutron beam; and lack of collaboration of medical team with research reactor centers, among others. Some of the recent BNCT studies in clinical trials worldwide are summarized in Table 2.2.

Table 2.2 Recent clinical trials on boron neutron capture therapy.

BNCT agent	Administration protocol	Malignancy	No. of patients	Irradiation dose	Country	Clinical trial phase	Status	Ref.
BPA	Interventional (500 mg/kg, 6/kg/h for 2 h before irradiation. During irradiation, BPA continued at 100 mg/kg/h.	Recurrent malignant gliomas	27	Scalp dose: 8.5 Gy-Eq	Japan	II	Completed	[125]
BPA	Interventional (500 mg/kg), 200 mg/kg/h for 2 h before irradiation. During irradiation, BPA continued at 100 mg/kg/h.	Head & neck cancer	21	Mucosa dose: 12 Gy-Eq	Japan	II	Completed/ post-marketing approval	[126]
BPAF	Interventional (290–500 mg/ kg)	Glioblastoma	50	NA	Finland	I and II	Terminated (slow accrual)	[127]
BPA	Interventional (500 mg/kg)	Recurrent high-grade meningiomas	18	Scalp dose: 7.5 Gy-Eq	Japan	II	Ongoing	[128]
BSH	Interventional/12–18 h before irradiation/repeated for 4 d	Glioblastoma multiforme	36	NA	Austria, Canada, France, Germany, Italy, The Netherlands, and European Organization for Research and Treatment of Cancer	I	Completed	[129]

(*Continued*)

Table 2.2 (*Continued*)

BNCT agent	Administration protocol	Malignancy	No. of patients	Irradiation dose	Country	Clinical trial phase	Status	Ref.
BPA	Interventional (500 mg/kg), 200 mg/kg/h for 2 h before irradiation. During irradiation, BPA continued at 100 mg/kg/h.	Malignant melanoma, angiosarcoma	9	NA	Japan	I	Ongoing	[130]
BPA	Interventional (350 mg/kg in 90 min)	Melanoma	NA	NA	China	I/II	Recruiting	[131]
BSH+BPA	Interventional, BSH 100 mg/kg/1 h/13 h before irradiation + Interventional, BPA (200–500 mg/kg for 2 h)	Glioblastoma multiforme	32	NA	Japan	II/ multicenter	Completed	[132]
^{18}F-BPA+BPA	Interventional/400 mg/m^2/2 h	Head & neck cancer	17	NA	Finland	I/II	Terminated	[133]
F-BPA	BPA-PET imaging	Solid tumor, adult	NA	NA	China	NA	Not yet recruiting	[134]
BPA	Interventional (500 mg/kg)	Recurrent malignant gliomas	27	Scalp dose: 8.5 Gy-Eq	Japan	II	Completed	[135]
sodium borocaptate	Interventional, adjuvant therapy	Brain and central nervous system tumors	36	NA	European Organization for Research and Treatment of Cancer	I	Completed	[136]

2.4 Conclusions and Perspectives

Why is it difficult to develop a boron carrier for BNCT? Clearly, from the enormous literature for the design and synthesis of boron delivery agents, it is not due to a lack of trying. However, until now only two drugs are used in clinics, *i.e.*, BPA and BSH. The challenge is much more difficult than the design of traditional tumor imaging agents and chemotherapeutics because, in contrast to radiopharmaceuticals, these agents must deliver a sufficient amount of ^{10}B to all tumor cells in order to sustain a lethal $^{10}B(n,\alpha)^7Li$ capture reaction. Moreover, they must persist for a sufficient amount of time in tumor cells and simultaneously clear from surrounding normal tissues. So far, various boron entities have been explored but all the works remain in preclinical studies without IND approval.

A significant hurdle remains in the form of a lack of convincing experimental animal data of boron delivery agents that could warrant the initiation of expensive clinical biodistribution studies. It is well recognized that the application of a new drug requires considerable experimental information such as active pharmaceutical ingredient (API) production, toxicology evaluation in at least one non-rodent animal species, and clinical studies in different phases. Secondly, scaling up synthesis is also a major challenge before clinical studies can be initiated. In addition, new drugs also need to be prepared in good manufacturing practice (GMP) facilities for clinical usage.

Moving forward, the following critical issues need to be addressed: (1) discovering more efficient and reliable boron agents, and (2) developing new methods to determine and quantitate the boron-10 concentration in tumors *in situ*. In Japan and Finland, the *in situ* analytical technology based on ^{18}F-BPA PET imaging is a well-established technique for the treatment of genital cancers [71, 140]. It remains to be seen whether the results would be sufficient to convince physicians across the world.

References

1. Barth, R. F., Coderre, J. A., Vicente, M. G. H. and Blue, T. E. (2005). Boron neutron capture therapy of cancer: current status and future prospects. *Clin. Cancer Res.* 11, 3987–4002.

2. Hawthorne, M. F. (1998). New horizons for therapy based on the boron neutron capture reaction. *Mol. Med. Today* **4**, 174–181.
3. Dai, Q., Yang, Q., Bao, X., Chen, J., Han, M. and Wei, Q. (2022). The development of boron analysis and imaging in boron neutron capture therapy (BNCT). *Mol. Pharm.* **19**, 363–377.
4. Armstrong, A. F. and Valliant, J. F. (2007). The bioinorganic and medicinal chemistry of carboranes: from new drug discovery to molecular imaging and therapy. *Dalton Trans.* **2007(38)**, 4240–4251.
5. Bregadze, V., Sivaev, I. and Glazun, S. (2006). Polyhedral boron compounds as potential diagnostic and therapeutic antitumor agents. *Anti-Cancer Agents Med. Chem.* **6**, 75–109.
6. Lesnikowski, Z. J. (2011). New Opportunities in Boron Chemistry for Medical Applications. In: Hosmane, N. S. (Ed.), *Boron Sciences: New Technologies and Applications*, CRC Press, pp. 3–19.
7. Valliant, J. F., Guenther, K. J., King, A. S., Morel, P., Schaffer, P., Sogbein, O. O. and Stephenson, K. A. (2002). The medicinal chemistry of carboranes. *Coord. Chem. Rev.* **232**, 173–230.
8. Leśnikowski, Z. J. (2016). Recent developments with boron as a platform for novel drug design. *Expert Opin. Drug Discov.* **11**, 569–578.
9. Adamska-Bartłomiejczyk, A., Bednarska, K., Białek-Pietras, M., Kiliańska, Z. M., Mieczkowski, A., Olejniczak, A. B., *et al.* (2018). Boron Cluster Modifications with Antiviral, Anticancer, and Modulation of Purinergic Receptors' Activities Based on Nucleoside Structures. In Hey-Hawkins, E. and Teixidor, C. V. (Eds.), *Boron-Based Compounds: Potential and Emerging Applications in Medicine*, John Wiley & Sons, pp. 20–34.
10. Hawthorne, M. F. and Maderna, A. (1999). Applications of radiolabeled boron clusters to the diagnosis and treatment of cancer. *Chem. Rev.* **99**, 3421–3434.
11. Qian, E. A., Wixtrom, A. I., Axtell, J. C., Saebi, A., Jung, D., Rehak, P., *et al.* (2017). Atomically precise organomimetic cluster nanomolecules assembled via perfluoroaryl-thiol SNAr chemistry. *Nat. Chem.* **9(4)**, 333–340.
12. Hawthorne, M. F. (1993). The role of chemistry in the development of boron neutron capture therapy of cancer. *Angew. Chem. Int. Ed. Eng.* **32**, 950–984.
13. Axtell, J. C., Saleh, L. M., Qian, E. A., Wixtrom, A. I. and Spokoyny, A. M. (2018). Synthesis and applications of perfunctionalized boron clusters. *Inorg. Chem.* **57(5)**, 2333–2350.
14. Hey-Hawkins, E. and Teixidor, C. V. (Eds.) (2018). *Boron-Based Compounds: Potential and Emerging Applications in Medicine.* John Wiley & Sons.
15. Zhu, Y., Lin, X., Xie, H., Li, J., Hosmane, N. S. and Zhang, Y. (2019). The current status and perspectives of delivery strategy for boron-based drugs. *Curr. Med. Chem.* **26**, 5019–5035.

16. Zhu, Y. and Hosmane, N. S. (2017). Ionic liquids: recent advances and applications in boron chemistry. *Eur. J. Inorg. Chem.* **2017**, 4369–4377.
17. Zhu, Y., Gao, S. and Hosmane, N. S. (2018). Boron-enriched advanced energy materials. *Inorg. Chim. Acta* **471**, 577–586.
18. Zhu, Y. and Hosmane, N. S. (2018). Nanostructured boron compounds for cancer therapy. *Pure Appl. Chem.* **90**, 653–663.
19. Barth, R. F., Zhang, Z. and Liu, T. (2018). A realistic appraisal of boron neutron capture therapy as a cancer treatment modality. *Cancer Commun.* **38**, 36.
20. Moss, R. L. (2014). Critical review, with an optimistic outlook, on boron neutron capture therapy (BNCT). *Appl. Radiat. Isot.* **88**, 2–11.
21. Körbe, S., Schreiber, P. J. and Michl, J. (2006). Chemistry of the carba-closo-dodecaborate (–) anion, CB11H12. *Chem. Rev.* **106**, 5208–5249.
22. Núñez, R., Tarrés, M. R., Ferrer-Ugalde, A., de Biani, F. F., and Teixidor, F. (2016). Electrochemistry and photoluminescence of icosahedral carboranes, boranes, metallacarboranes, and their derivatives. *Chem. Rev.* **116**, 14307–14378.
23. Núñez, R., Romero, I., Teixidor, F. and Viñas, C. (2016). Icosahedral boron clusters: a perfect tool for the enhancement of polymer features. *Chem. Soc. Rev.* **45**, 5147–5173.
24. Olid, D., Nunez, R., Vinas, C. and Teixidor, F. (2013). Methods to produce B–C, B–P, B–N and B–S bonds in boron clusters. *Chem. Soc. Rev.* **42**, 3318–3336.
25. Grimes, R. (2016). *Carboranes* (3rd ed.). Academic Press, 2016, pp. 945–984.
26. Hosmane, N. S. (2016). *Boron Science: New Technologies and Applications.* CRC Press.
27. Farr, L. E., Sweet, W. H., Locksley, H. B. and Robertson, J. S. (1954). Neutron capture therapy of gliomas using boron. *Trans. Am. Neurol. Assoc.* **13**(79th Meeting), 110–113.
28. Godwin, J. T., Farr, L. E., Sweet, W. H. and Robertson, J. S. (1955). Pathological study of eight patients with glioblastoma multiforme treated by neutron capture therapy using boron 10. *Cancer* **8**, 601–615.
29. Miyatake, S.-I., Kawabata, S., Hiramatsu, R., Kuroiwa, T., Suzuki, M., Kondo, N. and Ono, K. (2016). Boron neutron capture therapy for malignant brain tumors. *Neurol. Med. Chir. (Tokyo)* **56**, 361–371.
30. Chen, Y.-W., Lee, Y.-Y., Lin, C.-F., Pan, P.-S., Chen, J.-K., Wang, C.-W., et al. (2021). Salvage boron neutron capture therapy for malignant brain tumor patients in compliance with emergency and compassionate use: evaluation of 34 cases in Taiwan. *Biology* **10**(4), 334.
31. Miyatake, S.-I., Wanibuchi, M., Hu, N. and Ono, K. (2020). Boron neutron capture therapy for malignant brain tumors. *J. Neuro-oncol.* **149**, 1–11.
32. Kawabata, S., Suzuki, M., Hirose, K., Tanaka, H., Kato, T., Goto, H., et al. (2021). Accelerator-based BNCT for patients with recurrent glioblastoma: a multicenter phase II study. *Neuro-oncol. Adv.* **3**, vdab067.

33. Kusaka, S., Morizane, Y., Tokumaru, Y., Tamaki, S., Maemunah, I. R., Akiyama, Y., Sato, F. and Murata, I. (2022). Cerebrospinal fluid-based boron delivery system may help increase the uptake boron for boron neutron capture therapy in veterinary medicine: A preliminary study with normal rat brain cells. *Res. Veter. Sci.* **148**, 1–6.

34. Kankaanranta, L., Seppälä, T., Koivunoro, H., Saarilahti, K., Atula, T., Collan, J., *et al.* (2012). Boron neutron capture therapy in the treatment of locally recurred head-and-neck cancer: final analysis of a phase I/II trial. *Int. J. Radiat. Oncol. Biol. Phys.* **82**, e67–e75.

35. Koivunoro, H., Kankaanranta, L., Seppälä, T., Haapaniemi, A., Mäkitie, A. and Joensuu, H. (2019). Boron neutron capture therapy for locally recurrent head and neck squamous cell carcinoma: An analysis of dose response and survival. *Radiother. Oncol.* **137**, 153–158.

36. Suzuki, M., Sakurai, Y., Hagiwara, S., Masunaga, S., Kinashi, Y., Nagata, K., *et al.* (2007). First attempt of boron neutron capture therapy (BNCT) for hepatocellular carcinoma. *Japanese J. Clin. Oncol.* **37**, 376–381.

37. Yanagie, H., Higashi, S., Seguchi, K., Ikushima, I., Fujihara, M., Nonaka, Y., *et al.* (2014). Pilot clinical study of boron neutron capture therapy for recurrent hepatic cancer involving the intra-arterial injection of a ^{10}BSH-containing WOW emulsion. *Appl. Radiat. Isot.* **88**, 32–37.

38. Bakeine, G., Di Salvo, M., Bortolussi, S., Stella, S., Bruschi, P., Bertolotti, A., *et al.* (2009). Feasibility study on the utilization of boron neutron capture therapy (BNCT) in a rat model of diffuse lung metastases. *Appl. Radiat. Isot.* **67**, S332-S335.

39. Farías, R. O., Garabalino, M. A., Ferraris, S., Santa María, J., Rovati, O., Lange, F., *et al.* (2015). Toward a clinical application of ex situ boron neutron capture therapy for lung tumors at the RA-3 reactor in Argentina. *Med. Phys.* **42**, 4161–4173.

40. Trivillin, V. A., Serrano, A., Garabalino, M. A., Colombo, L. L., Pozzi, E. C., Hughes, A. M., *et al.* (2019). Translational boron neutron capture therapy (BNCT) studies for the treatment of tumors in lung. *Int. J. Radiat. Biol.* **95**, 646–654.

41. Andoh, T., Fujimoto, T., Suzuki, M., Sudo, T., Sakurai, Y., Tanaka, H., *et al.* (2015). Boron neutron capture therapy (BNCT) as a new approach for clear cell sarcoma (CCS) treatment: Trial using a lung metastasis model of CCS. *Appl. Radiat. Isot.* **106**, 195–201.

42. Suzuki, M., Endo, K., Satoh, H., Sakurai, Y., Kumada, H., Kimura, H., *et al.* (2008). A novel concept of treatment of diffuse or multiple pleural tumors by boron neutron capture therapy (BNCT). *Radiother. Oncol.* **88**, 192–195.

43. Suzuki, M., Sakurai, Y., Masunaga, S., Kinashi, Y., Nagata, K., Maruhashi, A. and Ono, K. (2007). A preliminary experimental study of boron neutron capture

therapy for malignant tumors spreading in thoracic cavity. *Japanese J. Clin. Oncol.* **37**, 245–249.

44. Suzuki, M., Sakurai, Y., Masunaga, S., Kinashi, Y., Nagata, K., Maruhashi, A. and Ono, K. (2006). Feasibility of boron neutron capture therapy (BNCT) for malignant pleural mesothelioma from a viewpoint of dose distribution analysis. *Int. J. Radiat. Oncol. Biol. Phys.* **66**, 1584–1589.

45. Masunaga, S.-I., Sakurai, Y., Tano, K., Tanaka, H., Suzuki, M., Kondo, N., *et al.* (2014). Effect of bevacizumab combined with boron neutron capture therapy on local tumor response and lung metastasis. *Exp. Ther. Med.* **8**, 291–301.

46. Masunaga, S.-I., Sakurai, Y., Tanaka, H., Takata, T., Suzuki, M., Sanada, Y., *et al.* (2019). Usefulness of combination with both continuous administration of hypoxic cytotoxin and mild temperature hyperthermia in boron neutron capture therapy in terms of local tumor response and lung metastatic potential. *Int. J. Radiat. Biol.* **95**, 1708–1717.

47. Farías, R. O., Bortolussi, S., Menéndez, P. R. and González, S. J. (2014). Exploring boron neutron capture therapy for non-small cell lung cancer. *Phys. Med.* **30**, 888–897.

48. Santa Cruz, G., Bertotti, J., Marín, J., González, S., Gossio, S., Alvarez, D., *et al.* (2009). Dynamic infrared imaging of cutaneous melanoma and normal skin in patients treated with BNCT. *Appl. Radiat. Isot.* **67**, S54-S58.

49. Menéndez, P., Roth, B., Pereira, M., Casal, M., González, S., Feld, D., *et al.* (2009). BNCT for skin melanoma in extremities: Updated Argentine clinical results. *Appl. Radiat. Isot.* **67**, S50-S53.

50. Zhang, Z., Yong, Z., Jin, C., Song, Z., Zhu, S., Liu, T., *et al.* (2020). Biodistribution studies of boronophenylalanine in different types of skin melanoma. *Appl. Radiat. Isot.* **163**, 109215.

51. Alberti, D., Deagostino, A., Toppino, A., Geninatti Crich, S. and Aime, S. (2019). Preclinical studies of MRI guided BNCT at Torino and Pavia Universities. In *Proceedings of the 38th Annual Meeting of the European Society for Radiotherapy and Oncology* (ESTRO), pp.307–308.

52. Lai, Z.-Y., Li, D.-Y., Huang, C.-Y., Tung, K.-C., Yang, C.-C., Liu, H.-M., Chou, F.-I. and Chuang, Y.-J. (2022). Valproic acid enhances radiosensitization via DNA double-strand breaks for boronophenylalanine-mediated neutron capture therapy in melanoma cells. *Anticancer Res.* **42**, 3413–3426.

53. Yuan, T. Z., Xie, S. Q. and Qian, C. N. (2019). Boron neutron capture therapy of cancer: Critical issues and future prospects. *Thoracic Cancer* **10**, 2195–2199.

54. Scholz, M. and Hey-Hawkins, E. (2011). Carbaboranes as pharmacophores: properties, synthesis, and application strategies. *Chem. Rev.* **111**, 7035–7062.

55. Jalilian, A. R., Shahi, A., Swainson, I. P., Nakamura, H., Venkatesh, M. and Osso, J. A. (2022). Potential theranostic boron neutron capture therapy agents as multimodal radiopharmaceuticals. *Cancer Biother. Radiopharm.* **37**, 342–354.

56. Hughes, A. M. (2022). Importance of radiobiological studies for the advancement of boron neutron capture therapy (BNCT). *Expert Rev. Mol. Med.* **24**, e14.

57. Ono, K., Kinashi, Y., Suzuki, M., Takagaki, M. and Masunaga, S. I. (2000). The combined effect of electroporation and borocaptate in boron neutron capture therapy for murine solid tumors. *Japan. J. Cancer Res.* **91**, 853–858.

58. Wada, Y., Hirose, K., Harada, T., Sato, M., Watanabe, T., Anbai, A., *et al.* (2018). Impact of oxygen status on 10B-BPA uptake into human glioblastoma cells, referring to significance in boron neutron capture therapy. *J. Radiat. Res.* **59**, 122–128.

59. Heber, E. M., Hawthorne, M. F., Kueffer, P. J., Garabalino, M. A., Thorp, S. I., Pozzi, E. C., *et al.* (2014). Therapeutic efficacy of boron neutron capture therapy mediated by boron-rich liposomes for oral cancer in the hamster cheek pouch model. *Proc. Natl. Acad. Sci.* **111**, 16077–16081.

60. Barth, R. F., Wu, G., Yang, W., Binns, P. J., Riley, K. J., Patel, H., *et al.* (2004). Neutron capture therapy of epidermal growth factor (+) gliomas using boronated cetuximab (IMC-C225) as a delivery agent. *Appl. Radiat. Isot.* **61**, 899–903.

61. Oleshkevich, E., Morancho, A., Saha, A., Galenkamp, K. M., Grayston, A., Crich, S. G., *et al.* (2019). Combining magnetic nanoparticles and icosahedral boron clusters in biocompatible inorganic nanohybrids for cancer therapy. *Nanomed. Nanotech. Biol. Med.* **20**, 101986.

62. Torresan, V., Guadagnini, A., Badocco, D., Pastore, P., Muñoz Medina, G. A., Fernàndez van Raap, M. B., *et al.* (2021). Biocompatible iron–boron nanoparticles designed for neutron capture therapy guided by magnetic resonance imaging. *Adv. Health. Mater.* **10**, 2001632.

63. Kawai, K., Nishimura, K., Okada, S., Sato, S., Suzuki, M., Takata, T. and Nakamura, H. (2020). Cyclic RGD-functionalized closo-dodecaborate albumin conjugates as integrin targeting boron carriers for neutron capture therapy. *Mol. Pharm.* **17**, 3740–3747.

64. Ban, H. S. and Nakamura, H. (2015). Boron-based drug design. *Chem. Record* **15**, 616–635.

65. Couto, M., Alamón, C., Nievas, S., Perona, M., Dagrosa, M. A., Teixidor, F., *et al.* (2020). Bimodal therapeutic agents against glioblastoma, one of the most lethal forms of cancer. *Chem. Eur. J.* **26**, 14335–14340.

66. Nuez-Martinez, M., Pinto, C. I., Guerreiro, J. F., Mendes, F., Marques, F., Muñoz-Juan, A., *et al.* (2021). Cobaltabis (dicarbollide)([o-COSAN]-) as multifunctional chemotherapeutics: a prospective application in boron neutron capture therapy (BNCT) for glioblastoma. *Cancers* **13(24)**, 6367.

67. Scott, J. G., Sedor, G., Ellsworth, P., Scarborough, J. A., Ahmed, K. A., Oliver, D. E., *et al.* (2021). Pan-cancer prediction of radiotherapy benefit using genomic-adjusted radiation dose (GARD): a cohort-based pooled analysis. *Lancet Oncol.* **22**, 1221–1229.

68. Sauerwein, W. A., Sancey, L., Hey-Hawkins, E., Kellert, M., Panza, L., Imperio, D., *et al.* (2021). Theranostics in boron neutron capture therapy. *Life* **11**, 330.
69. Ferrari, E., Wittig, A., Basilico, F., Rossi, R., De Palma, A., Di Silvestre, D., *et al.* (2019). Urinary proteomics profiles are useful for detection of cancer biomarkers and changes induced by therapeutic procedures. *Molecules* **24**, 794.
70. Watanabe, T., Hattori, Y., Ohta, Y., Ishimura, M., Nakagawa, Y., Sanada, Y., *et al.* (2016). Comparison of the pharmacokinetics between L-BPA and L-FBPA using the same administration dose and protocol: a validation study for the theranostic approach using [^{18}F]-L-FBPA positron emission tomography in boron neutron capture therapy. *BMC Cancer* **16**, 1–10.
71. Hiratsuka, J., Kamitani, N., Tanaka, R., Yoden, E., Tokiya, R., Suzuki, M., Barth, R. F. and Ono, K. (2018). Boron neutron capture therapy for vulvar melanoma and genital extramammary Paget's disease with curative responses. *Cancer Commun.* **38**(1), 38.
72. Teixidor, F. and Viñas C. (2018). Halogenated Icosahedral Carboranes: A Platform for Remarkable Applications. In: Hosmane, N. S. and Eagling, R. (Eds.), *Handbook Of Boron Science: With Applications In Organometallics, Catalysis, Materials And Medicine (In 4 Volumes).* World Scientific, pp. 205–228.
73. Rodriguez, C., Carpano, M., Curotto, P., Thorp, S., Casal, M., Juvenal, G., Pisarev, M. and Dagrosa, M. A. (2018). In vitro studies of DNA damage and repair mechanisms induced by BNCT in a poorly differentiated thyroid carcinoma cell line. *Radiat. Environ. Biophys.* **57**, 143–152.
74. Sato, A., Itoh, T., Imamichi, S., Kikuhara, S., Fujimori, H., Hirai, T., *et al.* (2015). Proteomic analysis of cellular response induced by boron neutron capture reaction in human squamous cell carcinoma SAS cells. *Appl. Radiat. Isot.* **106**, 213–219.
75. Kang, W., Svirskis, D., Sarojini, V., McGregor, A. L., Bevitt, J. and Wu, Z. (2017). Cyclic-RGDyC functionalized liposomes for dual-targeting of tumor vasculature and cancer cells in glioblastoma: An in vitro boron neutron capture therapy study. *Oncotarget* **8**, 36614.
76. Koning, G. A., Fretz, M. M., Woroniecka, U., Storm, G. and Krijger, G. C. (2004). Targeting liposomes to tumor endothelial cells for neutron capture therapy. *Appl. Radiat. Isot.* **61**, 963–967.
77. Ono, K., Masunaga, S. I, Kinashi, Y., Takagaki, M., Akaboshi, M., Suzuki, M. and Baba, H. (1998). Effects of boron neutron capture therapy using borocaptate sodium in combination with a tumor-selective vasoactive agent in mice. *Japan. J. Cancer Res.* **89**, 334–340.
78. Masunaga, S.-I., Sakurai, Y., Suzuki, M., Nagata, K., Maruhashi, A., Kinash, Y. and Ono, K. (2004). Combination of the vascular targeting agent ZD6126 with boron neutron capture therapy. *Int. J. Radiat. Oncol. Biol. Phys.* **60**, 920–927.

79. Yoneyama, T., Hatakeyama, S., Sutoh Yoneyama, M., Yoshiya, T., Uemura, T., Ishizu, T., et al. (2021). Tumor vasculature-targeted [10]B delivery by an Annexin A1-binding peptide boosts effects of boron neutron capture therapy. *BMC Cancer* **21**, 72.

80. Mukai, K., Nakagawa, Y. and Matsumoto, K. (1995). Prompt gamma ray spectrometry for in vivo measurement of boron-10 concentration in rabbit brain tissue. *Neurol. Med. Chir.* **35**, 855–860.

81. Barth, R. F., Adams, D. M., Soloway, A. H., Mechetner, E. B., Alam, F. and Anisuzzaman, A. K. (1991). Determination of boron in tissues and cells using direct-current plasma atomic emission spectroscopy. *Anal. Chem.* **63**, 890–893.

82. Michel, J., Sauerwein, W., Wittig, A., Balossier, G. and Zierold, K. (2003). Subcellular localization of boron in cultured melanoma cells by electron energy-loss spectroscopy of freeze-dried cryosections. *J. Microsc.* **210**, 25–34.

83. Basilico, F., Sauerwein, W., Pozzi, F., Wittig, A., Moss, R. and Mauri, P. (2005). Analysis of [10]B antitumoral compounds by means of flow-injection into ESI-MS/MS. *J. Mass Spectrom.* **40**, 1546–1549.

84. Bendel, P., Koudinova, N. and Salomon, Y. (2001). In vivo imaging of the neutron capture therapy agent BSH in mice using [10]B MRI. *Magn. Reson. Med.* **46**, 13–17.

85. Reifschneider, O., Schütz, C. L., Brochhausen, C., Hampel, G., Ross, T., Sperling, M. and Karst, U. (2015). Quantitative bioimaging of p-boronophenylalanine in thin liver tissue sections as a tool for treatment planning in boron neutron capture therapy. *Anal. Bioanal. Chem.* **407**, 2365–2371.

86. Aldossari, S., McMahon, G., Lockyer, N. P. and Moore, K. L. (2019). Microdistribution and quantification of the boron neutron capture therapy drug BPA in primary cell cultures of human glioblastoma tumour by NanoSIMS. *Analyst* **144**, 6214–6224.

87. Igaki, H., Murakami, N., Nakamura, S., Yamazaki, N., Kashihara, T., Takahashi, A., et al. (2022). Scalp angiosarcoma treated with linear accelerator-based boron neutron capture therapy: A report of two patients. *Clin. Transl. Radiat. Oncol.* **33**, 128–133.

88. Morita, T., Kurihara, H., Hiroi, K., Honda, N., Igaki, H., Hatazawa, J., et al. (2018). Dynamic changes in 18F-borono-L-phenylalanine uptake in unresectable, advanced, or recurrent squamous cell carcinoma of the head and neck and malignant melanoma during boron neutron capture therapy patient selection. *Radiat. Oncol.* **13**, 4.

89. Yokoyama, K., Miyatake, S.-I., Kajimoto, Y., Kawabata, S., Yoshida, T., Asano, T., et al. (2006). Pharmacokinetic study of BSH and BPA in simultaneous use for BNCT. *J. Neuro-oncol.* **78**, 227–232.

90. Amemiya, K., Takahashi, H., Kajimoto, Y., Nakazawa, M., Yanagie, H., Hisa, T., et al. (2005). High-resolution nuclear track mapping in detailed cellular histology

using CR-39 with the contact microscopy technique. *Radiat. Meas.* **40**, 283–288.

91. Wittig, A., Arlinghaus, H. F., Kriegeskotte, C., Moss, R. L., Appelman, K., Schmid, K. W. and Sauerwein, W. A. (2008). Laser postionization secondary neutral mass spectrometry in tissue: A powerful tool for elemental and molecular imaging in the development of targeted drugs. *Mol. Cancer Ther.* **7**, 1763–1771.

92. Arlinghaus, H., Spaar, M., Switzer, R. and Kabalka, G. (1997). Imaging of boron in tissue at the cellular level for boron neutron capture therapy. *Anal. Chem.* **69**, 3169–3176.

93. Kabalka, G. W., Davis, M. and Bendel, P. (1988). Boron-11 MRI and MRS of intact animals infused with a boron neutron capture agent. *Magn. Reson. Med.* **8**, 231–237.

94. Chandra, S., Barth, R. F., Haider, S. A., Yang, W., Huo, T., Shaikh, A. L., *et al.* (2013). Biodistribution and subcellular localization of an unnatural boron-containing amino acid (cis-ABCPC) by imaging secondary ion mass spectrometry for neutron capture therapy of melanomas and gliomas. *PLoS One* **8**, e75377.

95. Nakamura, H., Fukuda, H., Girald, F., Kobayashi, T., Hiratsuka, J., Akaizawa, T., *et al.* (2000). In vivo evaluation of carborane gadolinium-DTPA complex as an MR imaging boron carrier. *Chem. Pharma. Bull.* **48**, 1034–1038.

96. Ali, F., Hosmane, N. S. and Zhu, Y. (2020). Boron chemistry for medical applications. *Molecules* **25**, 828.

97. Singh, B., Kaur, G., Singh, P., Singh, K., Kumar, B., Vij, A., *et al.* (2016). Nanostructured boron nitride with high water dispersibility for boron neutron capture therapy. *Sci. Rep.* **6**, 35535.

98. Li, X., Wang, X. P., Zhang, J., Hanagata, N., Wang, X. B., Weng, Q. H., *et al.* (2017). Hollow boron nitride nanospheres as boron reservoir for prostate cancer treatment. *Nat. Commun.* **8**, 13936.

99. Ciofani, G., Raffa, V., Menciassi, A. and Cuschieri, A. (2008). Cytocompatibility, interactions, and uptake of polyethyleneimine-coated boron nitride nanotubes by living cells: Confirmation of their potential for biomedical applications. *Biotech. Bioeng.* **101**, 850–858.

100. Brokesh, A. M. and Gaharwar, A. K. (2020). Inorganic biomaterials for regenerative medicine. *ACS Appl. Mater. Interfaces* **12**, 5319–5344.

101. Emanet, C. M., Şen, O. Z. and Çulha, M. (2020). Hexagonal boron nitride nanoparticles for prostate cancer treatment. *ACS Appl. Nano Mater.* **3**, 2364–2372.

102. Hosmane, N. S., Maguire, J., Zhu, Y. and Takagaki, M. (Eds.) (2012). *Boron And Gadolinium Neutron Capture Therapy For Cancer Treatment.* World Scientific, pp. 165–170.

103. Vares, G., Jallet, V., Matsumoto, Y., Rentier, C., Takayama, K., Sasaki, T., *et al.* (2020). Functionalized mesoporous silica nanoparticles for innovative

boron-neutron capture therapy of resistant cancers. *Nanomed. Nanotech. Biol. Med.* **27**, 102195.

104. Wu, C.-Y., Hsieh, H.-H., Chang, T.-Y., Lin, J.-J., Wu, C.-C., Hsu, M.-H., *et al.* (2021). Development of MRI-detectable boron-containing gold nanoparticle-encapsulated biodegradable polymeric matrix for boron neutron capture therapy (BNCT). *Int. J. Mol. Sci.* **22**, 8050.

105. Wu, C.-Y., Lin, J.-J., Chang, W.-Y., Hsieh, C.-Y., Wu, C.-C., Chen, H.-S., *et al.* (2019). Development of theranostic active-targeting boron-containing gold nanoparticles for boron neutron capture therapy (BNCT). *Colloids Surf. B* **183**, 110387.

106. Das, B. C., Ojha, D. P., Das, S. and Evans, T. (2018). Boron Compounds in Molecular Imaging. In Hey-Hawkins, E. and Teixidor, C. V. (Eds.), *Boron-Based Compounds: Potential and Emerging Applications in Medicine*, John Wiley & Sons, pp. 205–231.

107. Tabbakh, F. and Hosmane, N. S. (2020). Enhancement of radiation effectiveness in proton therapy: Comparison between fusion and fission methods and further approaches. *Sci. Rep.* **10**, 5466.

108. Tsurubuchi, T., Shirakawa, M., Kurosawa, W., Matsumoto, K., Ubagai, R., Umishio, H., *et al.* (2020). Evaluation of a novel boron-containing -D-mannopyranoside for BNCT. *Cells* **9**, 1277.

109. Kalot, G., Godard, A., Busser, B., Pliquett, J., Broekgaarden, M., Motto-Ros, V., Wegner, K.D., Resch-Genger, U., Köster, U. and Denat, F. Aza-BODIPY: A new vector for enhanced theranostic boron neutron capture therapy applications. *Cells* **2020**, *9*, 1953.

110. Futamura, G., Kawabata, S., Nonoguchi, N., Hiramatsu, R., Toho, T., Tanaka, H., *et al.* (2017). Evaluation of a novel sodium borocaptate-containing unnatural amino acid as a boron delivery agent for neutron capture therapy of the F98 rat glioma. *Radiat. Oncol.* **12**, 26.

111. Li, J., Sun, Q., Lu, C., Xiao, H., Guo, Z., Duan, D., *et al.* (2022). Boron encapsulated in a liposome can be used for combinational neutron capture therapy. *Nat. Commun.* **13**, 2143.

112. Hattori, Y., Ishimura, M., Ohta, Y., Takenaka, H., Kawabata, S. and Kirihata, M. (2022). Dodecaborate conjugates targeting tumor cell overexpressing translocator protein for boron neutron capture therapy. *ACS Med. Chem. Lett.* **13**, 50–54.

113. Molinari, A. J., Thorp, S. I., Portu, A. M., Saint Martin, G., Pozzi, E. C., Heber, E. M., *et al.* (2015). Assessing advantages of sequential boron neutron capture therapy (BNCT) in an oral cancer model with normalized blood vessels. *Acta Oncol.* **54**, 99–106.

114. Garabalino, M. A., Olaiz, N., Portu, A., Saint Martin, G., Thorp, S. I., Pozzi, E. C., *et al.* (2019). Electroporation optimizes the uptake of boron-10 by tumor for boron neutron capture therapy (BNCT) mediated by GB-10: a boron biodistribution study in the hamster cheek pouch oral cancer model. *Radiat. Environ. Biophys.* **58**, 455–467.

115. Yamatomo, N., Iwagami, T., Kato, I., Masunaga, S.-I., Sakurai, Y., Iwai, S., *et al.* (2013). Sonoporation as an enhancing method for boron neutron capture therapy for squamous cell carcinomas. *Radiat. Oncol.* **8**, 280.

116. Lin, Y.-C., Chou, F.-I., Liao, J.-W., Liu, Y.-H. and Hwang, J.-J. The effect of low-dose gamma irradiation on the uptake of boronophenylalanine to enhance the efficacy of boron neutron capture therapy in an orthotopic oral cancer model. *Radiat. Res.* **195**, 347–354.

117. Kinashi, Y., Sakurai, Y., Masunaga, S., Takagaki, M. and Ono, K. (2001). Sensitizing effect of the phosphatidylinositol 3-kinase inhibitor wortmannin on thermal neutron irradiation with or without boron compound. *Radiat. Med.* **19**, 27–32.

118. Qi, P., Chen, Q., Tu, D., Yao, S., Zhang, Y., Wang, J., *et al.* (2020). The potential role of borophene as a radiosensitizer in boron neutron capture therapy (BNCT) and particle therapy (PT). *Biomater. Sci.* **8**, 2778–2785.

119. Perona, M., Rodríguez, C., Carpano, M., Thomasz, L., Nievas, S., Olivera, M., *et al.* (2013). Improvement of the boron neutron capture therapy (BNCT) by the previous administration of the histone deacetylase inhibitor sodium butyrate for the treatment of thyroid carcinoma. *Radiat. Environ. Biophys.* **52**, 363–373.

120. Conway-Kenny, R., Ferrer-Ugalde, A., Careta, O., Cui, X., Zhao, J., Nogués, C., *et al.* (2021). Ru (II) and Ir (III) phenanthroline-based photosensitisers bearing o-carborane: PDT agents with boron carriers for potential BNCT. *Biomater. Sci.* **9**, 5691–5702.

121. Tatebe, H., Masunaga, S.-I. and Nishimura, Y. (2020). Effect of rapamycin on the radio-sensitivity of cultured tumor cells following boron neutron capture reaction. *World J. Oncol.* **11**, 158–164.

122. Trivillin, V. A., Pozzi, E. C., Colombo, L. L., Thorp, S. I., Garabalino, M. A, Monti Hughes, A., *et al.* (2017). Abscopal effect of boron neutron capture therapy (BNCT): proof of principle in an experimental model of colon cancer. *Radiat. Environ. Biophys.* **56**, 365–375.

123. Trivillin, V. A., Langle, Y. V., Palmieri, M. A., Pozzi, E. C., Thorp, S. I., Benitez Frydryk, D. N., *et al.* (2021). Evaluation of local, regional and abscopal effects of Boron Neutron Capture Therapy (BNCT) combined with immunotherapy in an ectopic colon cancer model. *Brit. J. Radiol.* **94**, 20210593.

124. Marfavi, A., Kavianpour, P. and Rendina, L.M. (2022). Carboranes in drug discovery, chemical biology and molecular imaging. *Nat. Rev. Chem.* **6**, 486–504.

125. Fischli, W., Leukart, O. and Schwyzer, R. (1997). Hormone-receptor interactions. Carboranylalanine (Car) as a phenylalanine analogue: reactions with chymotrypsin. *Helv. Chim. Acta* **60**, 959–963.

126. Kongsbak, M., Levring, T. B., Geisler, C. and Von Essen, M. R. (2013). The vitamin D receptor and T cell function. *Front. Immunol.* **4**, 148.

127. Sirajudeen, S., Shah, I. and Al Menhali, A. (2019). A narrative role of vitamin D and its receptor: with current evidence on the gastric tissues. *Int. J. Mol. Sci.* **20**, 3832.

128. Hirose, K., Konno, A., Hiratsuka, J., Yoshimoto, S., Kato, T., Ono, K., *et al.* (2021). Boron neutron capture therapy using cyclotron-based epithermal neutron source and borofalan (^{10}B) for recurrent or locally advanced head and neck cancer (JHN002): An open-label phase II trial. *Radiother. Oncol.* **155**, 182–187.
129. https://jrct.niph.go.jp/en-latest-detail/jRCT2051190044.
130. https://www.clinicaltrials.jp/cti-user/trial/ShowDirect.jsp?japicId=JapicCTI-194742.
131. Miyatake, S.-I., Wanibuchi, M., Kawabata, S., Ko, N. and Ono, K. (2020). CTNI-56 — A phase II clinical trial using accelerator-based BNCT system for refractory recurrent high-grade meningioma. *Neuro Oncol.* **22**, ii55.
132. https://www.clinicaltrials.jp/cti-user/trial/ShowDirect.jsp?japicId=JapicCTI-194640.
133. https://clinicaltrials.gov/ct2/show/NCT04293289.
134. https://clinicaltrials.gov/ct2/show/NCT02759536.
135. https://clinicaltrials.gov/ct2/show/NCT00974987.
136. https://clinicaltrials.gov/ct2/show/NCT00927147.
137. https://clinicaltrials.gov/ct2/show/NCT05538676.
138. Miyatake, S-.I., *et al.* (2020). CTNI-26 — Accelerator-based BNCT in rescue treatment of patients with recurrent GBM: a multicenter phase II study. *Neuro Oncol.* **22**, 22, ii48.
139. https://clinicaltrials.gov/ct2/show/NCT00004015.
140. Kabalka, G. W., Smith, G. T., Dyke, J. P., Reid, W. S., Longford, C. D., Roberts, T. G., *et al.* (1997). Evaluation of fluorine-18-BPA-fructose for boron neutron capture treatment planning. *J. Nucl. Med.* **38**, 1762–1767.

https://doi.org/10.1142/9789811268038_0003

Chapter 3

Dendritic and Nanostructured Boron Compounds for Boron Neutron Capture Therapy

Soumya Sagar Dey,[1] Hiren Patel,[2] Narayan Hosmane[1,*]

[1]*Department of Chemistry and Biochemistry, Northern Illinois University, USA*
[2]*Department of Pathology, University of Illinois, USA*

Abstract

Boron-conjugated polymers are the most promising of the polymeric systems studied, especially since some polymer–drug conjugate therapies like PEGylated Doxorubicin have previously been licensed. While more research and insights are required for the most part, some studies are quite encouraging, particularly in terms of clinical translatability. FDA has approved a variety of nanoparticle delivery routes, with an emphasis on the intravenous route, which has advantages in the treatment of metastasized tumors. Because of their biodegradable and biocompatible behavior inside the human body, polymeric nanoparticles are garnering increased interest for the treatment of malignant gliomas. Over the years, a wide range of drugs have been synthesized to improve boron administration for boron neutron capture therapy (BNCT). Numerous small molecules were synthesized from natural products that provided a better tumor-to-blood ratio of boron in the *in vivo* studies. In the same way, many macromolecules have been synthesized with various secondary functions. This chapter will describe some of the dendrimers and nanoparticles developed for BNCT.

---

* Corresponding author.

Keywords: Boron neutron capture therapy, drug delivery, dendrimer, nanoparticle, biodegradable polymer.

3.1 Introduction to Boron Neutron Capture Therapy

In 1935, Chadwick and Goldhaber observed that low molecular weight nuclei such as boron could absorb slow neutrons [1]. Once the boron-10 (^{10}B) nucleus captures a neutron, the newly energized boron-11 undergoes a fission process [^{10}B(n, α)^{7}Li], producing an alpha and a lithium particle (Figure 3.1, left). Subsequently, Locher proposed using boron neutron capture (BNC) to treat cancer in 1936 [2]. Boron neutron capture therapy (BNCT) offers many benefits compared to conventional radiotherapy. BNCT utilizes non-ionizing slow neutron particles, reducing radiation's side effects. Since the BNC reaction only occurs in the presence of ^{10}B, the fission process will only take place in cells containing ^{10}B. Furthermore, the ionizing particles generated by these reactions travel a distance shorter than the radius of a cell, affecting only cancer cells housing ^{10}B, leaving healthy cells unharmed. As a result, systemic and local side effects can be minimized by selectively delivering ^{10}B to cancer cells.

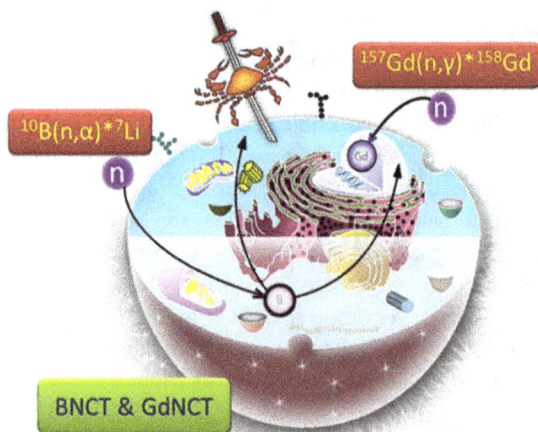

Figure 3.1   A schematic representation of boron and gadolinium neutron capture therapy.

With previous advantages in mind, the first *in vivo* studies using the BNC reaction were performed at the University of Illinois in 1938 [3]. Following a decade of laboratory experiments, the first patient received treatment at the Brookhaven National Laboratory (BNL) in 1951 with BNCT [4]. In these clinical trials at BNL, patients with malignant glioma were treated with variable doses of ^{10}B in the form of borax. Although none of the patients exhibited any severe adverse effects, failure to show substantial life extension resulted in the suspension of BNCT clinical trials in the U.S. A number of factors led to the failure of the trials at BNL. The primary reason is the lack of boron-containing molecules that can selectively target cancer cells. Various polyhedral boranes were tested in subsequent years at Mass General Hospital (MGH) to improve the BNC response. Due to low toxicity and ability to penetrate the blood-brain barrier, sodium mercapto-undecahydrododecaborate (BSH) was selected as an agent in the first BNCT clinical trials in Japan in 1968 [4]. Subsequently, another potent boron delivery agent, a derivative of phenylalanine called p-carboxy-phenyl-boronic acid (BPA) with low toxicity and higher capacity to penetrate into the central nervous system (CNS), was introduced.

Early clinical trials of BNCT focused on treating CNS tumors, primarily glioblastoma multiforme (GBM). Due to the low availability of surgical interventions and the limited number of chemotherapy drugs,

---

A case report [4]: Case-13 is of particular interest because BNCT apparently arrested the growth of his malignant cerebral tumor. A ~ 4 cm diameter carcinoma was removed from his anterior parietal region at a left temporoparietal craniotomy. Seven weeks later, a six-week course of cobalt-60 gamma radiation therapy (51 Gy to the whole brain) was begun. Recurrence of neurological signs, including right hemiparesis, led the patient to undergo BNCT at the Brookhaven Medical Research Reactor (BMRR). Six months after the termination of cobalt-60 therapy. The patient developed right hemiplegia, acute increased intracranial pressure, and a slight drop in systemic blood pressure (150/90-110/60 mmHg) about 10 h after BNCT. Following emergency treatment with intravenous urea, the patient slowly recovered and became ambulatory within 10 days. Before he left BNL 53 days later, not only had the paresis largely disappeared but remarkable

---

(Continued)

improvements in speech, ability to read, and vision were observed in comparison with the serious deficits in these functions (right hemiparesis, complete expressive aphasia, complete right homonymous hemianopia) that developed before BNCT. The patient did not deteriorate neurologically thereafter, but he died at BNL, severely jaundiced, five months after BNCT with widespread extracranial metastases, probably from a primary anaplastic carcinoma originating in the head of the pancreas (autopsy no. A-151-61; BNL). At necropsy, there was no evidence of viable brain tumor tissue or of brain edema.

GBM is difficult to treat. Table 3.1 outlines the GBM clinical trials in all facilities. A comparison of clinical data indicated that BNCT was superior to radiotherapy (RT) and radiotherapy/temozolomide (TMZ). Median survival time (MeST) from diagnosis for RT or RT/TMZ was 12.1 and 14.6 months, respectively [5], while for patients receiving BNCT with BPA or BSH, MeST was 16 and 23.3 months, respectively. Additionally, the quality of life of patients treated with RT and/or TMZ patients is also inferior to that of BNCT patients. Likewise, clinical trials for other tumors, including head and neck, melanoma, lung cancer, etc., using BNCT were conducted with great success.

Over the years, a wide range of drugs has been synthesized to improve boron administration for BNCT treatment. Numerous small molecules were synthesized from natural products that provided a better tumor-to-blood ratio of boron in the *in vivo* studies [9]. In the same way, many macromolecules have been synthesized with various secondary functions. This chapter will describe some of the dendrimers and nanoparticles developed for BNCT.

3.2 Introduction to Nanomaterials and Dendrimers

The term "nanoscale materials" refers to a group of substances with at least one dimension of fewer than 100 nanometers. Nanomaterials are fascinating because they exhibit unique optical, magnetic, electrical, and other properties at such a small scale. These emergent features could have huge implications in electronics, health, and other domains. Engineered

Table 3.1 BNCT clinical trials using epithermal neutron beams for patients with brain tumor [6–8].

Medical institution	Treatment dates	Tumor type and no. of patients	Boron compound and treatment	Clinical outcome
University of Tsukuba	1999–2002	5 GBM 4 AA	BSH 100 mg/kg in 1–1.5 h IO-BNCT	MeST: 23.2 mos (GBM) MeST: 25.9 mos (AA)
	1998–2007	7 GBM	BSH 5 g in 1 h, IO-BNCT	MeST: 23.3 mos 2 y OS: 43%
	1998–2007	8 GBM	BSH 5 g in 1 h and BPA 250 mg/kg in 1 h BNCT+XRT	MeST: 27.1 mos 2 y OS: 63%
University of Tokushima	1998–2000	6 GBM	BSH 64.9–178.6 mg/kg IO-BNCT	MeST: 15.5 mos 2 y OS: 0%
	2001–2004	11 GBM	BSH 64.9–178.6 mg/kg IO-BNCT	MeST: 19.5 mos 2 y OS: 27%
	2005–2008	6 GBM	BSH 100 mg/kg and BPA 250 mg/kg in 1 h or BSH 100 mg/kg and BPA 700 mg/kg in 6 h BNCT+XRT	MeST: 26.2 mos 2 y OS: 50%
Osaka Medical College	2002–2003	10 GBM	BSH 5 g and BPA 250 mg/kg in 1 h	MeST: 14.5 mos 2 y OS: 20%
	2003–2006	11 GBM	BSH 5 g and BPA 700 mg/kg in 6 h BNCT+XRT	MeST: 23.5 mos 2 y OS: 27.3%
	2002–2007	19 rGBM, 2 rAA, 1 rAOA	BSH 100 mg/kg and BPA 250 mg/kg in 1 h or BSH 100 mg/kg and BPA 700 mg/kg in 6 h	MeST: 10.8 mos post-BNCT 2 y OS: 14%
	2010–2013	32 nGBM	BSH 5 g/body in 1 h + BPA 500 mg/kg in 3 h (BNCT + XRT + TMZ)	21.1 mos (2 yr OS: 45.5%)
	2013–2018	10 rGBM	BPA 500 mg/kg in 3 h (BNCT + Bev)	12 mos

(*Continued*)

Table 3.1 (*Continued*)

Medical institution	Treatment dates	Tumor type and no. of patients	Boron compound and treatment	Clinical outcome
Brookhaven National Laboratory, Upton, NY, USA	1994–1999	53 nGBM	BPA 250–330 mg/kg in 2 h	12.8 mos
Beth Israel Deaconess Medical Center, Harvard Medical School, Boston, USA	1996–1999 2002–2003	20 nGBM 6 nGBM	BPA 250–350 mg/kg in 1.5 h BPA 14 g/m2 in 1.5 h	11.1 mos NA
Universitätsklinikum Essen, Essen, Germany	1997–2002	26 nGBM	BSA 100 mg/kg in 1.7 h	10.4–13.2 mos
Helsinki University Central Hospital, Helsinki, Finland	1999–2001 2001–2008	30 nGBM 20 rGBM	BPA 290–500 mg/kg in 2 h BPA 290–450 mg/kg in 2 h	11.0–21.9 mos 7 mos (post-BNCT)
Faculty Hospital of Charles University, Prague, Czech Republic	2000–2002	5 nGBM	BSH 100 mg/kg in 1 h	NA
Nyköping Hospital, Nyköping, Sweden	2001–2003 2001–2005	29 nGBM 12 rGBM	BPA 900 mg/kg in 6 h BPA 900 mg/kg in 6 h	17.7 mos 8.7 mos (post-BNCT)

Including other disease sites and patients treated off-protocol, the total number of patients treated at some reactors is much greater than reported here: for FiR-1, ~260, for KURR, >107, and for JRR-4, >200 patients.

Treatment is indicated only in cases when it is not solely external beam BNCT.

Abbreviations: n newly diagnosed, r recurrent, GBM glioblastoma multiforme, IC MM intracranial metastatic melanoma, AA anaplastic astrocytoma, MMng malignant meningioma, MC mesenchymal chondrosarcoma, AOA anaplastic oligoastrocytoma, MRM meningioma related malignancy, IO-BNCT intraoperative BNCT, XRT external beam radiation therapy (photons), MeST median survival time, 2 y OS 2 year overall survival , RI

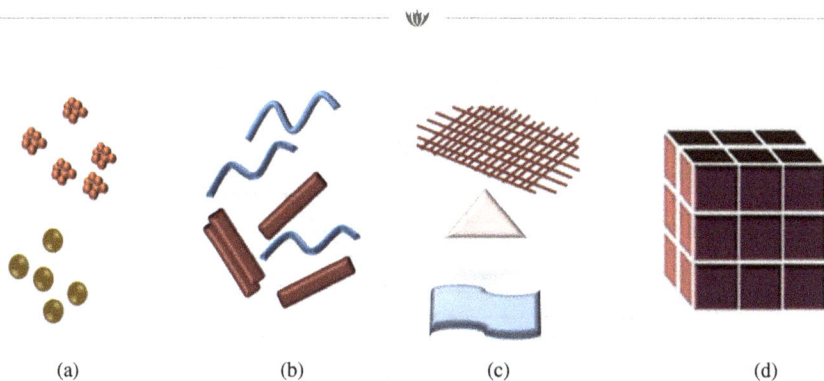

(a)   (b)   (c)   (d)

Figure 3.2 Classification of nanomaterials [11]. (a) 0D spheres and clusters. (b) 1D nanofibers, wires, and roads. (c) 2D films, plates, and networks. (d) 3D nanomaterials.

nanomaterials are resources that have been developed at the molecular level to take advantage of their small size and unique features that are not found in their bulk counterparts [10]. Increased relative surface area and novel quantum effects are the two fundamental reasons materials at the nanoscale might have distinct characteristics. Nanomaterials can be nanoscale in one dimension (*e.g.*, surface films), two dimensions (*e.g.*, strands or fibers), or three dimensions (*e.g.*, particles) [11]. They can exist in single, fused, aggregated, or agglomerated forms with spherical, tubular, and irregular shapes. Common types of nanomaterials include nanotubes, nanosheets, nanowires, and nanorods (Figure 3.2).

In zero-dimensional nanomaterials, all the dimensions are measured within the nanoscale (no dimensions are larger than 100 nm). In one-dimensional nanomaterials, one dimension is outside the nanoscale. This class includes nanotubes, nanorods, and nanowires. In two-dimensional nanomaterials, two dimensions are outside the nanoscale. This class exhibits plate-like shapes and includes graphene, nanofilms, nanolayers, and nanocoatings. Three-dimensional nanomaterials are materials that are not confined to the nanoscale in any dimension. This class can contain bulk powders, dispersions of nanoparticles, bundles of nanowires and nanotubes as well as multi-nanolayers [12].

Dendrimers are synthetic nanoscale compounds that have unique properties which make them useful in the medical and pharmaceutical industries. Dendrimers are radially symmetric, nanoscale molecules with a well-defined, homogenous, and monodisperse structure made up of tree-like arms or branches [13]. Fritz Vogtle was the first to identify

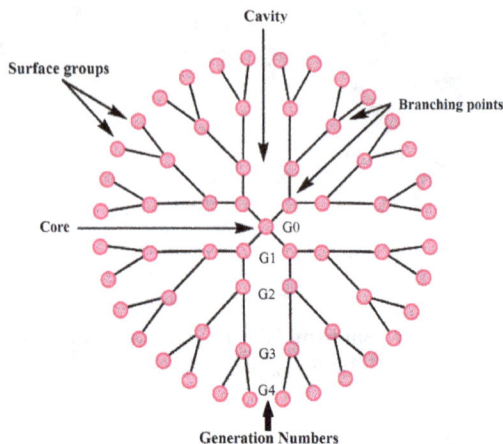

Figure 3.3 Structure of a dendrimer [21]. From central structure to periphery, 0–4 generations.

these hyperbranched compounds in 1978. Dendrimers are macromolecules that are essentially monodisperse and have symmetric branching units constructed around a small molecule or linear polymer core [14]. A dendrimer consists of an inner initiator core, followed by several repeating interior layers and an exterior surface with multiple active groups [15,16].

They are synthesized by stacking layers of branching groups on top of each other where each new layer is referred to as a generation (Figure 3.3). Hence, dendrimers are distinguished by their 'generation', which is the number of branching cycles performed during synthesis and is proportional to their size [17]. In the final generation, surface molecules will give the dendrimer the desired function for pharmaceutical, life science, chemical, electronic, and materials applications [13].

3.3 Advantages of Nanomaterials and Dendrimers

Nanomaterials have a large surface area-to-volume ratio, which aids in drug loading. Hundreds of pharmacological molecules can be encapsulated in a single polymeric nanomaterial. They have also been employed in drug transporting, gene delivery, pathogen and protein bio-detection,

DNA structure probing, tissue engineering, tumor detection, and purification of biological molecules [18]. Nanomedicine is the use of nanomaterials in medicine. Nanomedicine encompasses everything from medicinal nanomaterials and biological devices to nanoelectronic biosensors and, potentially in the future, molecular nanotechnology applications such as biological machines. The long-term goal of nano-medicine research is nanomachinery. When a magnetic field is applied externally, these nanoparticles spin [19]. Theranostic nanomaterials undergo easy surface modification and hence possess a high drug-loading capacity for numerous small-molecule anticancer drugs, enzymes, and therapeutic genes [20]. The application of dendrimers as a drug delivery system started in the late 1990s. Since their inception, dendrimers have been regarded as potential drug delivery vehicles due to their nanometric size and their ability to resolve issues with poor solubility, toxicity, or stability when combined with other drugs [21]. There are three main reasons that justify the use of dendrimers for drug delivery [22]. The presence of multiple copies of a drug may cause a multivalency effect, similar to the polyvalent interactions that are common in biological systems [23]. Solubility is an important asset in chemistry. Dendrimer-based formulations may improve solubility and thus bioavailability [24]. In addition, dendrimers are often used in biology and nanomedicine research due to their controllable and adjustable size (generally several nanometers), which exceeds the renal threshold and is not filtered out by the kidneys. Their nanometric size may result in the enhanced penetration and retention (EPR) effect [25,26].

Owing to the above structural and chemical properties, dendrimers find application as drug delivery agents [27], carriers or scaffolds for diagnosis [28], contrasting agents for MRI [29], tissue generators [30] and in development of vaccines [31]. There are numerous instances of medications conjugated with dendrimers, with the main goal of boosting specificity at the site of action while reducing systemic toxicity by directing distribution to the tumor cell. Poly(amidoamine) dendrimers (PAMAM, Figure 3.4) have been frequently conjugated with various drugs like Doxorubicin for lung cancer and brain tumor [32], Paclitaxel and Docetaxel for breast cancer [33], 5-fluorouracil for gastric

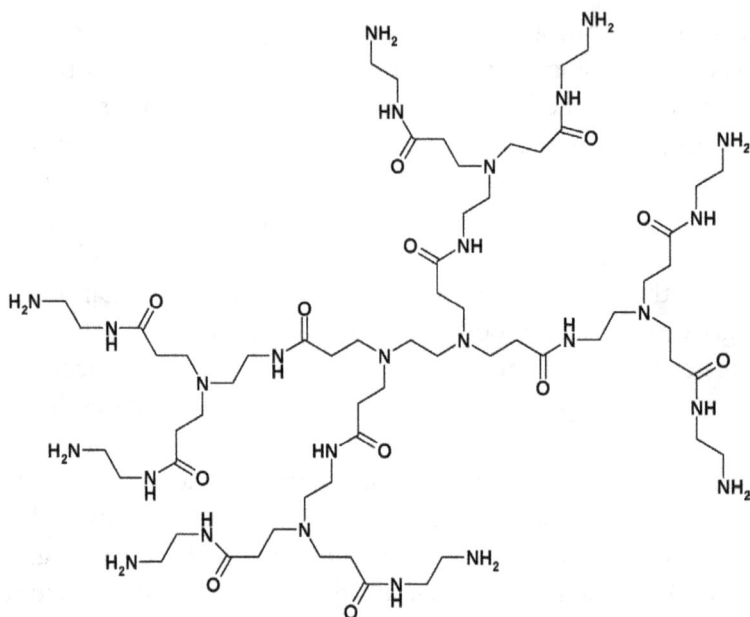

Figure 3.4   Chemical structure of PAMAM dendrimer, generation 1 (or G1) [32].

neoplasm [34], Sunitinib for renal neoplasm [35] and Cisplatin for breast and ovarian neoplasm [36].

3.4 BNCT for Treatment of Cancer

To modify the planned therapy, it is vital to study and investigate the dimension and several other aspects of the malignant tissue. The detection, accurate localization, and quantification of ^{10}B in sick tissues to guide radiation treatment are very crucial in BNCT [37–39]. Therefore, the development of small molecules that can be used for therapeutic and diagnostic purposes *in vivo*, so-called theranostic agents, is highly important. BNCT is a treatment method that combines chemotherapy and conventional radiation. While the selective concentration of boron compounds in tumor cells can improve the effect of neutron beam radiation [40], BNCT may fail due to the non-specificity of the boron delivery agents, the presence of boron delivery agents in excessive concentrations in the blood, and an insufficient radiation dose [41]. For therapeutic purposes, the medications should be tumor-selective and allow for high boron accumulation in cancer cells, as well as possess all other qualities necessary for BNCT treatments. This cancer treatment is not currently widely available, and the indications for its use are limited. BNCT has been used to treat the following cancers so far: extramammary Paget's disease [42], GBM [43], head and neck cancer [44], multifocal hepatocellular carcinoma [45], recurrent lung cancer [46], squamous cell carcinomas, salivary gland carcinomas, sarcomas, and recurrent malignant meningioma [47].

3.4.1 Glioblastoma Multiforme

Despite full resection, radiation, and adjuvant chemotherapy [48], GBM remains one of the most difficult cancers to cure. GBM, also known as grade IV glioma, is the most frequent malignant brain tumor in adults, according to the World Health Organization. It has a very poor prognosis, and there is an urgent need to improve patient stratification and treatment [41]. The restricted penetrability of the blood-brain barrier (BBB), resistance to standard therapy, and inadequate DNA repair capability all contribute to the difficulty of treating glioblastoma. As a result, BNCT has been proposed as a treatment option in the upfront and recurrent settings. Boron has been shown to possess direct tumoricidal activity and can cross the BBB [49]. Unfortunately, the clinical findings obtained by various organizations have not indicated that BNCT is an effective treatment for glioblastoma [51–54]. There has been interest in combining proton radiation and BNCT as the usage of protons has expanded. In a short trial, patients who received BNCT with proton treatment had a greater survival rate than those who received radiation plus temozolomide; however, the difference was not statistically significant [50]. According to the European Organization for Research and Treatment of Cancer, the best treatment results are achieved when postoperative photon irradiation is combined with temozolomide administration, and only effective and newly developed delivery drugs suitable for clinical trials can change this paradigm.

3.4.2 *Head and Neck Cancer*

Squamous cell carcinoma of the head and neck (HNSCC), often known as head and neck cancer, is a prevalent malignant cancer with a high death and morbidity rate [55]. HNSCC causes roughly 650,000 cases and 330,000 deaths each year around the world. It is treated with surgery, radiation, and platinum-based chemotherapy. The sole FDA-approved targeted therapy for head and neck cancer is cetuximab, a monoclonal antibody that targets EGFR; however, it has shown poor efficacy due to the establishment of resistance [56]. HNSCC is also frequently radio- and chemo-resistant and BNCT could be a generic answer to this issue. Although the bulk of clinical trials involving BNCT in head and neck cancers looked at it as a recurrent treatment, it has also been utilized as a final treatment. *In vitro*, BNCT suppresses oral SCC cells in both p53-dependent and p53-independent ways [57]. BNCT's efficacy against HNSCC has recently been established in several clinical trials, with an overall response rate of up to 90% [58–60]. Despite this, recurrence is common because of the non-homogeneous distribution of BPA in tumors [59].

3.4.3 *Melanoma*

Melanoma is a malignancy that is aggressive in humans and accounts for over 60% of all deadly skin cancers. Melanomas develop when DNA damage to skin cells is not repaired, resulting in mutations that lead to cell proliferation. Nodular melanoma, acral lentiginous melanoma, lentigo maligna, and superficial spreading melanoma are the different forms of melanoma [41]. Melanoma develops as a result of the combination of external and endogenous risk factors. Melanoma incidence has risen dramatically in both men and women over the last two decades [61], while it has been demonstrated to have a significant level of genomic instability [62]. Despite receiving the best treatment, patients with melanoma frequently have a bad prognosis. Surgical excision is the main treatment for melanoma. When the tumor has spread to other parts of the body, however, these treatments are ineffective. BNCT was first used to treat malignant melanoma with BPA in 1987 [63]. Outside of the CNS, this was the first time BNCT had been used. Despite identical histopathologic diagnoses, patients with melanoma treated with the same BNCT procedures can have variable clinical outcomes [64]. Because melanomas have the capacity to spread, both immuno-therapy and BNCT may be advised for treatment.

3.4.4 Malignant Mesothelioma

BNCT has been proposed for diffuse, unresectable lung tumors [65], as well as for inoperable malignant pleural mesothelioma [66–68]. Malignant mesothelioma (MM) is a rare and deadly cancer with a bleak outlook. Because MM is difficult to treat as it spreads easily, multimodal therapy is indicated. Surgery is useful in the early stages of the disease. The presence of many radiosensitive tissues reduces the efficiency of traditional radiation and limits the maximal dose [69]. Due to a lack of highly specific molecular markers, no effective targeted therapy exists, limiting the potential of an early MM diagnosis [45]. BNCT is a prom-ising treatment for inoperable patients due to their age or the presence of other illnesses [70]. The feasibility of treating shallow lung tumors with BNCT was confirmed in one study, although the role of BNCT in treating deeper tumors remains unknown [71].

3.4.5 BNCT for Prostate Cancer

In the treatment of prostate cancer, dose escalation utilizing external beam irradiation has been shown to be helpful in producing satisfactory, long-term outcomes. The best radiation method for treatment, on the other hand, is still a point of contention. The use of BNCT as a therapy option for localized, advanced prostate cancer is being discussed. The benefits of BNCT with BPA include preferential accumulation into tumor cells and augmentation of a highly localized dosage to the tumor cells without the risk of sub-lethal damage recovery lowering the irradiation's efficiency [72]. BNCT therapy is a treatment technique that avoids collateral radiation damage to healthy tissues in the sur-rounding area. Enough boron must therefore be collected within the tumor cell to generate a reasonable increase in cell death by BNCT. Several *in vivo* tests were carried out to find the best conditions for BPA accumulation inside the cell. In BPA-treated cells, acceptable values were determined [73]. The methods utilized to boost BPA uptake in cells, such as pH titration to dissolve BPA in HBSS (sickle cell anemia) and pre-treatment of cells with HBSS, are not suited for treating human patients. Alternative approaches, such as utilizing fructose complexed to BPA, are known to help solubilize BPA and allow for optimal BPA uptake in tumors [74]. BPA-fructose has become the most frequently used clinical boron delivery drug for both intra- and extra-cranial tumors [39]. *In vivo* cells exposed to 6 mM BPA or fewer showed no signs of drug toxicity, regardless of the length of exposure. Treatment of the cells with a higher quantity of BPA was shown to have negligible harmful effects. Treatment with BPA for a longer period of time and at a greater dose lowered clonogenic survival to 73% [74]. In additional research, BPA IC_{50} values for B-16 melanoma cells and TIG-1–20 normal human fetal lung hydro blast cells were found to be 8.6 and 2.2 mM, respectively [75].

The studies mentioned above show that a BNC reaction improves cell death in prostate cancer cells. Some issues must be resolved before clinical studies of BNCT for prostate cancer patients can commence. Neutron capture is one of them because neutrons can only reach organs close to the body's surface, and their effect diminishes as depth increases. As a result, even if BPA is properly delivered to prostate cancer cells, BNCT is unlikely to be effective if the prostate is neutron-irradiated from a normal direction. The distance between the prostate and the body surface would be significantly shortened if neutrons could be given transperineally [76].

3.4.6 BNCT for Treatment of Brain Cancer

The primary use of BNCT is in the treatment of malignant brain tumors such as GBM, as surgery is rarely able to remove all of the cancerous tissue; it is virtually untreatable and is inevitably lethal. Radiation- and chemotherapy-resistant cells remain dormant for long months following treatment, but eventually re-enter the cell cycle, leading to tumor regrowth. BNCT is a high-dose tumor-selective radiotherapy, which utilizes the non-radioactive isotope boron-10 (^{10}B) to capture thermal neutrons with a high probability leading to the nuclear reaction of

$^{10}B(n,\alpha)^7Li$ [77]. Previous research [78] has shown that proliferative cells targeted for thermal neutron death absorb ^{10}B. Unfortunately, a lack of effective absorption of existing boron agents by glioma stem cells (GSCs) leads to glioma cell survival and tumor recurrence after BNCT. As a result, a crucial requirement for successful BNCT is the development of new formulations for boron medicines that target GSCs.

Many dendrimer-based techniques have been used to improve the uptake of boron-10 in GSCs. In a recent study [79], an amine dendrimer linked to CD133 monoclonal antibodies was produced, encapsulating BSH, and the uptake of the bioconjugate nanoparticles by GSCs *in vitro* and *in vivo* was monitored. PAMAM was used as the dendrimer. *In vitro*, more than 90% of CD133+ cells absorbed PD-CD133/BSH compared to less than 40% of CD133 cells. Similar uptake of PD-CD133/BSH to CD133+ cells was also seen in animal models. These findings suggest that delivering PD-CD133/BSH to specific cells promotes cellular uptake and therapeutic efficacy. Mice injected with BSH-encapsulating boron lipid liposomes at a dose of 15 mg B/kg had a high boron content and substantial anticancer effect after thermal neutron irradiation. In glioma-implanted mice, the survival statistics with the combination PAMAM-CD133/BSH with BSH were superior to those given single BSH (Table 3.2). The mean survival time of mice implanted with CD133+-SU2 glioma xenografts exposed to PAMAM-CD133/BSH in combination with BSH was 61.8 days after neutron irradiation, compared to 46.7 days in mice implanted with CD133-SU2 glioma xenografts, 45.9 days with BSH alone, and 35.8 days with PAMAM-CD133. A single mouse lived >90 days in the PAMAM-CD133/BSH paired with BSH plus BNCT group, which was considered prolonged survival.

Because of their biological applications in targeted drug delivery, thermotherapy, and contrast enhancement in magnetic resonance imaging, magnetic nanoparticles (MNPs) have gotten a lot of interest. In a small number of *in vivo* investigations using functional MNPs as drug transporters, promising findings have been obtained. The reduction of the required number of cytotoxic drugs, as well as the related side effects, is a major benefit of this technology. This method has been

Table 3.2   Radiation dosages in various groups of SU2 and U87 cells [79].

Cell lines	Group		Time (min)					
			5	10	15	20	25	30
SU2	Neutron radiation (CD133+ cells)	$^{10}B(n,\alpha)^7$ Li	—	—	—	—	—	—
		total dosage	0.083	0.166	0.249	0.332	0.415	0.498
	BSH (CD133+ cells)	$^{10}B(n,\alpha)^7Li$	0.047	0.094	0.141	0.188	0.235	0.282
		total dosage	0.130	0.260	0.390	0.520	0.650	0.780
	PD-CD133/BSH (CD133− cells)	$^{10}B(n,\alpha)^7Li$	0.111	0.222	0.333	0.444	0.555	0.666
		total dosage	0.194	0.388	0.582	0.776	0.970	1.164
	PD-CD133/BSH (CD133+ cells)	$^{10}B(n,\alpha)^7Li$	0.503	1.006	1.509	2.012	2.515	3.018
		total dosage	0.586	1.172	1.758	2.344	2.930	3.516
U87s	Neutron radiation (CD133+ cells)	$^{10}B(n,\alpha)^7Li$	—	—	—	—	—	—
		total dosage	0.083	0.166	0.249	0.332	0.415	0.498
	BSH (CD133+ cells)	$^{10}B(n,\alpha)^7Li$	0.041	0.082	0.123	0.164	0.205	0.246
		total dosage	0.124	0.248	0.372	0.496	0.620	0.744
	PD-CD133/BSH (CD133− cells)	$^{10}B(n,\alpha)^7Li$	0.105	0.210	0.315	0.420	0.525	0.630
		total dosage	0.188	0.376	0.564	0.752	0.940	1.128
	PD-CD133/BSH (CD133+ cells)	$^{10}B(n,\alpha)^7Li$	0.486	0.972	1.458	1.944	2.430	2.916
		total dosage	0.569	1.138	1.707	2.276	2.845	3.414

tested for targeting cytotoxic medications to brain tumors. Particles as large as 1–2 μm have been shown to be localized at the site of intracerebral rat glioma-2 tumors in studies [80]. Commercially available magnetic nanoparticles of iron oxides matrixed with starch enriched with carborane cages exhibited excellent accumulation in tumor cells in high concentration in the presence of an external magnetic field. Studies conducted in BALB/c mice showed that boron concentrations in the tumor were less than 14.7 μg/g tumor at various time intervals, with slow clearance after 30 hours, in the absence of an external magnetic field. This is lower than that in *nido*-carborane-attached water-soluble single-walled carbon nanotubes, which had a maximum boron concentration of 22.8 μg/g tumor after 30 hours. The highest concentration of 51.4 μg/g tumor was achieved in the presence of an external magnetic field, with tumor/normal tissue ratios of roughly 10:1. These results show that the delivery system could be used to treat not only brain tumors but also other types of cancers using BNCT [81].

Phenylene-cored dendrimers with three, six, or nine peripheral o-carborane clusters are another similar technique. After 20 hours of incubation, *in vitro* biological evaluation of the dendrimer containing nine carborane units revealed that it accumulated in human hepato-cellular carcinoma cells or was bound to their surface, with a boron concentration of up to 2540 ng per 5×10^5 cells. Such a concentration amounts to around 1.5 mg of boron per gram of tumor that, when adjusted for the natural abundance of ^{10}B, yields a value of 300 µg/g, which is more than the 30 µg of ^{10}B per g of tumor required for effective BNCT and hence this technique can be extended to glial cells [82].

Microbubbles (MBs) and transcranial-focused ultrasound (FUS) have been shown to open the BBB/BTB at the target position non-invasively and reversibly, creating a temporary time window for improving therapeutic drug delivery into brain tissue [83]. MBs can also serve as carriers for low molecular weight drugs in a variety of ways, including hydrophobic interaction to keep hydrophobic drugs in the MBs, electrostatic interaction to attach charged molecules (*e.g.*, DNA and RNA) to cationic shells on MBs, and covalent coupling to attach biomolecules to MB shells. This strategy could help cytotoxic chemotherapy medicines. A novel anionic block copolymer, poly(ethylene glycol) conjugated with BSH (PEG-b-PMBSH) of size 300 nm, containing MBs (B-MBs) coupled with FUS showed effective accumulation in tumor sites by EPR effect. MB-assisted FUS treatment for GBM therapy showed no brain damage resulting from high BTB permeability. From the specific acoustic intensity, the BTB opening effect was confirmed to continue for as long as 1 hour. Boron uptake was verified to increase with increasing FUS irradiation time, while brain damage was only observed with longer irradiation treatment. It was observed that PEG-b-PMBSH had high drug delivery efficiency (7.1%) as compared to previously reported studies. After FUS irradiation, the combination of PEG-b-PMBSH and MBs (B-MBs) did not result in considerable boron uptake in the tumor immediately, but steadily increased over time. PEG-b-PMBSH has a long blood circulation and, as a result of the EPR effect, is more likely to boost tumor uptake. The boron compounds had poor distribution in other organs and were promptly removed *via* numerous mechanisms [84]. These results provide new hope for a combination of the drugs with BNCT/MRI/thermotherapy.

Folate receptor (FR) expression is increased in a number of human malignancies while being restricted in the majority of normal tissues [85]. The brain, lung, and certain sarcomas are among the FR-overexpressing malignancies that may be treated with neutron capture therapy. Endocytosis mediated by FR transports folic acid (FA) into cells. Polyethylene glycol (PEG) modification of a wide range of molecules has been reported, including low molecular weight medicines, proteins, liposomes, and viruses. Improved aqueous solubility, longer blood circulation due to reduced renal and reticuloendothelial system clearance, as well as lower enzymatic degradation and toxicity, are a few advantages of PEGylated compounds. Based on this success, FA-conjugated and non-conjugated PEGylated carborane-appended PAMAM derivatives have been studied *in vitro* using FR+ cells and *in vivo* using a murine tumor model [86]. The compound with the highest number of boron clusters and short PEG chain showed the highest percentage of uptake per gram of liver (34%) in C57BL/6 mice. Similar results were obtained *in vitro* where the derivative with the highest number of boron clusters and short PEG showed double the cellular uptake as compared to others. In fact, bio-distribution studies also showed higher tumor uptake for the PEGylated carborane-appended PAMAM derivative having the highest number of boron clusters.

Intravenous injection of BSH with PEGylated polyglutamic acid, or PEG-b-P(Glu-BSH), was administered to BALB/c mice bearing subcutaneous implants of the Colon-26 (C26) cancer cell line (Figure 3.5). After a single intravenous injection of 50 mg/kg, a tumor-to-blood ratio of 20:1 and 70–90 g of ^{10}B per gram of tumor were recorded. *In vivo* BNCT was carried out after 24 hours of intravenous injection of PEG-b-P(Glu-BSH) into tumor-bearing animals. Glu-BSH appeared

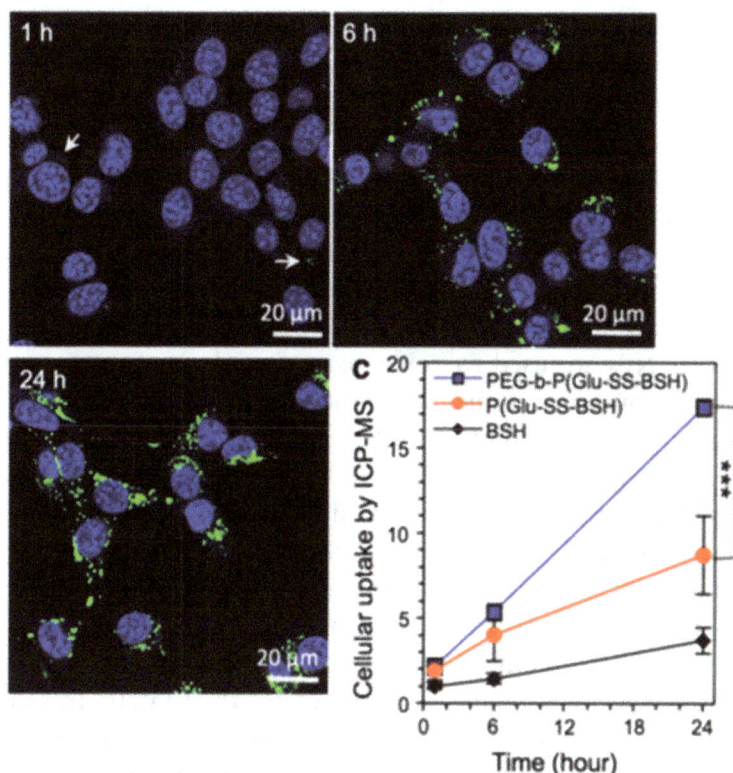

Figure 3.5 Time-lapsed cellular uptake of PEG-b-P(Glu-SS-BSH) by C26 cancer cells was investigated by confocal laser scanning microscope. Both PEG-b-P(Glu-SS-BSH) and P(Glu-SS-BSH) were labeled with Alexa488 (green), and their dose was stained with Hoechst (blue) [35].

to be superior to BSH, as demonstrated by higher tumor-to-normal tissue and tumor-to-blood ratios [86].

3.5 Conclusion

It can be concluded that boron-conjugated polymers are the most promising of the polymeric systems studied, especially since some polymer-drug conjugate therapies like PEGylated Doxorubicin have previously been licensed [87]. In the last three years, many strategies to improve targeted drug delivery *via* nanoparticles (NPs) have been proposed. While more research and insights are required for the most part, some studies are quite promising, particularly in terms of clinical translatability. Combined treatments and NP functionalization can meet many needs for various cell types, and even well-known medications can be repurposed. This emphasizes the prospect of designing tailor-made treatments for each patient using nanomedicine, thereby corroborating precision and personalized medicine at the same time. The number of different ways for designing NPs is practically infinite. Sometimes NPs are used to compensate for a lack of response from free medications, for instance when the available drugs are polar molecules and cannot permeate inside target cells [88]. On the other hand, the design of a specific NP could be tweaked to improve drug responsiveness. For example, many individuals with solid tumors do not react to CAR-T cell treatments [89]. This is due to the fact that solid tumors can restrict T-cell activity by secreting inhibitory substances into the tumor microenvironment. Biomimetics is a viable tool due to its inherent properties, such as the ability to replicate existing biological structures and so increase their safety. In fact, the negative effects of these medicines can be much decreased, and numerous varieties of these biomimetic NPs can theoretically be created. Non-spherical NPs also outperform spherical NPs in cell interactions and crossing biological barriers. As a result, this discovery may point to more effective techniques for improving drug delivery. The FDA has approved various NP delivery routes, with an emphasis on the intravenous route, which has advantages in treating metastasized tumors [90].

Because of their biodegradable and biocompatible behavior inside the human body, polymeric NPs are garnering interest for the treatment of malignant gliomas. The path to creating a suitable system, however, is not easy, especially for polymer-small drug conjugates, where the EPR effect appears to be crucial. As a result, although having a system with adequate boron is one condition, ensuring that this system reaches only the targeted cell in sufficient quantities is another. Labeling and targeting moieties will undoubtedly be important considerations in the development of successful BNCT carriers. More work is needed to optimize the size, drug loading capacity, and release of hydrophilic and hydrophobic drugs conjugated with nanomaterials, taking into account the many physicochemical and physiological hurdles that could stymie their success. Finally, in the coming years, the main goal should be to avoid the flaws of these unique approaches and to improve therapy translatability.

References

1. Chadwick, J. and Goldhaber, M. (1935). Disintegration by slow neutrons. *Math. Proc. Cambridge Philos. Soc.* **31**, 612–616.
2. Locher, G. L. (1936). Biological effects and therapeutic possibilities of neutrons. *Am. J. Roentgenol.* **36**, 1–13.
3. Kruger, P. G. (1940). Some biological effects of nuclear disintegration products on neoplastic tissue. *Proc. Natl. Acad. Sci.* **26**, 181–192.
4. Slatkin, D. N. (1991). A history of boron neutron capture therapy of brain tumors. *Brain* **114**, 1609–1629.
5. Sander, A., Wosniok, W. and Gabel, D. (2014). Case numbers for a randomized clinical trial of boron neutron capture therapy for glioblastoma multiforme. *Appl. Radiat. Isot.* **88**, 16–19.
6. Miyatake, S. I., Kawabata, S., Hiramatsu, R., Kuroiwa, T., Suzuki, M., Kondo, N., *et al.* (2016). Boron neutron capture therapy for malignant brain tumors. *Neurol. Med. Chir. (Tokyo)* **56**, 361–371.
7. Barth, R. F., Vicente, M. G. H., Harling, O. K., Kiger III, W. S., Riley, K. J., Binns, P. J., *et al.* (2012). Current status of boron neutron capture therapy of high grade gliomas and recurrent head and neck cancer. *Radiat. Oncol.* **7**, 146.
8. Hideghéty, K., Brunner, S., Cheesman, A., Szabó, E. R., Polanek, R., Margarone, D., *et al.* (2019). Boron delivery agents for boron proton-capture enhanced proton therapy. *Anticancer Res.* **39**, 2265–2276.
9. Hosmane, N. S. (Ed.) (2016). *Boron Science: New Technologies and Applications.* CRC Press.
10. Albalawi, F., Hussein, M. Z., Fakurazi, S. and Masarudin, M. J. (2021). Engineered nanomaterials: The challenges and opportunities for nanomedicines. *Int. J. Nanomed.* **16**, 161–184.
11. Trotta, F. and Mele, A. (Eds.) (2019). *Nanosponges: Synthesis and Applications.* John Wiley & Sons, pp. 1–26.
12. Abdullaeva, Z. (2017). *Nano- and Biomaterials: Compounds, Properties, Characterization, and Applications.* John Wiley & Sons, pp. 27–56.
13. Abbasi, E., Aval, S. F., Akbarzadeh, A. Milani, M. and Nasrabadi, H. T. (2014). Dendrimers: synthesis, applications, and properties. *Nanoscale Res. Lett.* **9**, 247.

14. Kopecký, D. and Škodová, J. (2014). Laser induced transfer of organic materials. *J. Opt. Res.* **16**, 47–72.
15. Kesharwani, P., Jain, K. and Jain, N. K. (2014). Progress in polymer science dendrimer as nanocarrier for drug delivery. *Prog. Polym. Sci.* **39**, 268–307.
16. Duncan, R. and Izzo, L. (2005). Dendrimer biocompatibility and toxicity. *Adv. Drug Deliv. Rev.* **57**, 2215–2237.
17. Mishra, V. and Kesharwani, P. (2016). Dendrimer technologies for brain tumor. *Drug Discov. Today* **21**, 766–778.
18. Zdrojewicz, Z., Waracki, M., Bugaj, B., Pypno, D. and Cabała, K. (2015). Medical applications of nanotechnology zastosowanie nanotechnologii w medycynie. *Postepy Hig. Med. Dosw.* **69**, 1196–1204.
19. Saha, M. (2009). Nanomedicine: promising tiny machine for the healthcare in future-a review. *Oman Med. J.* **24**, 242–247.
20. Raja, I. S., Kang, M. S., Kim, K. S., Jung, Y. J.and Han, D.-W. (2020). Two-dimensional theranostic nanomaterials in cancer treatment: state of the art and perspectives. *Cancers (Basel)* **12**, 1657.
21. Aurelia Chis, A., Dobrea, C., Morgovan, C., Arseniu, A. M., Rus, L. L., Butuca, A., *et al.* (2020). Applications and limitations of dendrimers in biomedicine. *Molecules* **25**, 3982.
22. Caminade, A. M. and Turrin, C. O. (2014). Dendrimers for drug delivery. *J. Mater. Chem. B* **2**, 4055–4066.
23. Mammen, M., Choi, S. K. and Whitesides, G. M. (1998). Polyvalent interactions in biological systems: implications for design and use of multivalent ligands and inhibitors. *Angew. Chem. Int. Ed.* **37**, 2754–2794.
24. Jain, N. K. and Tekade, R. K. (2013). Dendrimers for Enhanced Drug Solubilization. In: Douroumis, D. and Fahr, A. (Eds.), *Drug Delivery Strategies for Poorly Water-Soluble Drugs*, John Wiley & Sons, pp. 373–409.
25. Maeda, H., Miyamoto, Y., Seymour, L. W. and Seymour, L. W. (1992). Conjugates of anticancer agents and polymers: advantages of macromolecular therapeutics in vivo. *Bioconjug. Chem.* **3**, 351–362.
26. Maeda, H., Wu, J., Sawa, T., Matsumura, Y. and Hori, K. (2000). Tumor vascular permeability and the EPR effect in macromolecular therapeutics: a review. *J. Control. Release* **65**, 271–284.
27. Madaan, K., Kumar, S., Poonia, N., Lather, V. and Pandita, D. (2014). Dendrimers in drug delivery and targeting: drug-dendrimer interactions and toxicity issues. *J. Pharm. Bioallied Sci.* **6**, 139–150.
28. Gupta, U., Dwivedi, S. K. D., Bid, H. K., Konwar, R. and Jain, N. K. (2010). Ligand anchored dendrimers based nanoconstructs for effective targeting to cancer cells. *Int. J. Pharm.* **393**, 186–197.
29. Liu, M. and Fréchet, J. M. (1999). Designing dendrimers for drug delivery. *Pharm. Sci. Technolo. Today* **2**, 393–401.
30. Joshi, N. and Grinstaff, M. (2008). Applications of dendrimers in tissue engineering. *Curr. Top. Med. Chem.* **8**, 1225–1236.

31. Heegaard, P. M. H., Boas, U. and Sorensen, N. S. (2010). Dendrimers for vaccine and immunostimulatory uses. A review. *Bioconjug. Chem.* **21**, 405–418.

32. Borkowski, T., Subik, P., Trzeciak, A. M. and Wołowiec, S. (2011). Palladium(0) deposited on PAMAM dendrimers as a catalyst for C-C cross coupling reactions. *Molecules* **16**, 427–441.

33. Kesharwani, P., Tekade, R. K., Gajbhiye, V., Jain, K. and Jain, N. K. (2011). Cancer targeting potential of some ligand-anchored poly(propylene imine) dendrimers: a comparison. *Nanomed.* **7**, 295–304.

34. Entezar-Almahdi, E., Mohammadi-Samani, S., Tayebi, L. and Farjadian, F. (2020). Recent advances in designing 5-fluorouracil delivery systems: a stepping stone in the safe treatment of colorectal cancer. *Int. J. Nanomed.* **15**, 5445–5458.

35. Adams, V. R. and Leggas, M. (2007). Sunitinib malate for the treatment of metastatic renal cell carcinoma and gastrointestinal stromal tumors. *Clin. Ther.* **29**, 1338–1353.

36. Duan, X., He, C., Kron, S. J. and Lin, W. (2016). Nanoparticle formulations of cisplatin for cancer therapy. *WIREs Nanomed. Nanobiotechnol.* **8**, 776–791.

37. Burnet, N. G., Thomas, S. J., Burton, K. E. and Jefferies, S. J. (2004). Defining the tumor and target volumes for radiotherapy. *Cancer Imaging* **4**, 153–161.

38. Malouff, T. D., Seneviratne, D. S., Ebner, D. K., Stross, W. C., Waddle, M. R., Trifiletti, D. M., *et al.* (2021). Boron neutron capture therapy: a review of clinical applications. *Front. Oncol.* **11**, 601820.

39. Sauerwein, W. A. G., Sancey, L., Hey-Hawkins, E., Kellert, M., Panza, L., Imperio, D., *et al.* (2021). Theranostics in boron neutron capture therapy. *Life (Basel)* **11**, 330.

40. Hawthorne, M. F. (1993). The role of chemistry in the development of boron neutron capture therapy of cancer. *Angew. Chem. Int. Ed.* **32**, 950–984.

41. Dymova, M. A., Taskaev, S. Y., Richter, V. A. and Kuligina, E. V. (2020). Boron neutron capture therapy: current status and future perspectives. *Cancer Commun.* **40**, 406–421.

42. Hiratsuka, J., Kamitani, N., Tanaka, R., Yoden, E., Tokiya, R. and Suzuki, M. (2018). Boron neutron capture therapy for vulvar melanoma and genital extramammary Paget's disease with curative responses. *Cancer Commun.* **38**, 38.

43. Miyatake, S. I., Kawabata, S., Hiramatsu, R., Kuroiwa, T., Suzuki, M. and Ono, K. (2018). Boron neutron capture therapy of malignant gliomas. *Prog. Neurol. Surg.* **32**, 48–56.

44. Wang, L. W., Wan, Y., Liu, H., Chou, F. I. and Jiang, S. H. (2018). Clinical trials for treating recurrent head and neck cancer with boron neutron capture therapy using the Tsing — Hua open pool reactor. *Cancer Commun.* **38**, 1–7.

45. Yanagie, H., Higashi, S., Seguchi, K., Ikushima, I., Fujihara, M., Nonaka, Y., *et al.* (2014). Pilot clinical study of boron neutron capture therapy for recurrent hepatic cancer involving the intra-arterial injection of a ^{10}BSH-containing WOW emulsion. *Appl. Radiat. Isot.* **88**, 32–37.

46. Suzuki, M., Suzuki, O., Sakurai, Y., Tanaka, H., Kondo, N., Kinashi, Y., *et al.* (2012). Reirradiation for locally recurrent lung cancer in the chest wall with boron neutron capture therapy (BNCT). *Int. Canc. Conf. J.* 1, 235–238.
47. Koivunoro, H., Kankaanranta, L., Seppälä, T., Haapaniemi, A., Mäkitie, A. and Joensuu, H. (2019). Boron neutron capture therapy for locally recurrent head and neck squamous cell carcinoma: an analysis of dose response and survival. *Radiother. Oncol.* 137, 153–158.
48. Stupp, R., Mason, W. P., van den Bent, M. J., Weller, M., Fisher, B., Taphoorn, M. J. B., *et al.* (2005). Radiotherapy plus concomitant and adjuvant temozolomide for glioblastoma. *N. Engl. J. Med.* 352, 987–996.
49. Altinoz, M. A., Topcu, G. and Elmaci, İ. (2019). Boron's neurophysiological effects and tumoricidal activity on glioblastoma cells with implications for clinical treatment. *Int. J. Neurosci.* 129, 963–977.
50. Sköld, K., Gorlia, T., Pellettieri, L., Giusti, V., H-Stenstam, B. and Hopewell, J. W. (2010). Boron neutron capture therapy for newly diagnosed glioblastoma multiforme: an assessment of clinical potential. *Br. J. Radiol.* 83, 596–603.
51. Miyatake, S.-I., Kawabata, S., Kajimoto, Y., Aoki, A., Yokoyama, K., Yamada, M., *et al.* (2005). Modified boron neutron capture therapy for malignant gliomas performed using epithermal neutron and two boron compounds with different accumulation mechanisms: an efficacy study based on findings on neuroimages. *J. Neurosurg.* 103, 1000–1009.
52. Miyatake, S.-I., Kawabata, S., Yokoyama, K., Kuroiwa, T., Michiue, H., Sakurai, Y., *et al.* (2009). Survival benefit of boron neutron capture therapy for recurrent malignant gliomas. *J. Neurooncol.* 91, 199–206.
53. Kawabata, S., Miyatake, S., Kuroiwa, T., Yokoyama, K., Doi, A., Iida, K., *et al.* (2009). Boron neutron capture therapy for newly diagnosed glioblastoma. *J. Radiat. Res.* 50, 51–60.
54. Kankaanranta, L., Seppälä, T., Koivunoro, H., Välimäki, P., Beule, A., Collan, J., *et al.* (2011). L-Boronophenylalanine-mediated boron neutron capture therapy for malignant glioma progressing after external beam radiation therapy: A phase I study. *Int. J. Radiat. Oncol. Biol. Phys.* 80, 369–376.
55. Jou, A. and Hess, J. (2017). Epidemiology and molecular biology of head and neck cancer. *Oncol. Res. Treat.* 40, 328–332.
56. Leonard, B., Brand, T. M., O'Keefe, R. A., Lee, E. D., Zeng, Y., Kemmer, J. D., *et al.* (2018). BET inhibition overcomes receptor tyrosine kinase–mediated cetuximab resistance in HNSCC. *Cancer Res.* 78, 4331–4343.
57. Fujita, Y., Kato, I., Iwai, S., Ono, K., Suzuki, M., Sakurai, Y., *et al.* (2009). Role of p53 mutation in the effect of boron neutron capture therapy on oral squamous cell carcinoma. *Radiat. Oncol.* 4, 63.
58. Aihara, T., Morita, N., Kamitani, N., Kumada, H., Ono, K., Hiratsuka, J., *et al.* (2014). BNCT for advanced or recurrent head and neck cancer. *Appl. Radiat. Isot.* 88, 12–15.

59. Haapaniemi, A., Kankaanranta, L., Saat, R., Koivunoro, H., Saarilahti, K., Mäkitie, A., *et al.* (2016). Boron neutron capture therapy in the treatment of recurrent laryngeal cancer. *Int. J. Radiat. Oncol. Biol. Phys.* **95**, 404–410.

60. Kankaanranta, L., Seppälä, T., Koivunoro, H., Saarilahti, K., Atula, T., Collan, J., *et al.* (2012). Boron neutron capture therapy in the treatment of locally recurred head-and-neck cancer: final analysis of a phase I/II trial. *Int. J. Radiat. Oncol. Biol. Phys.* **82**, e67–e75.

61. Jemal, A., Ward, E. M., Johnson, C. J., Cronin, K. A., Ma, J., Ryerson, B., *et al.* (2017). Annual report to the nation on the status of cancer, 1975–2014, featuring survival. *J. Natl. Cancer Inst.* **109**, djx030.

62. Martincorena, I. and Campbell, P. J. (2016). Erratum for the review "Somatic mutation in cancer and normal cells" by *Science* **351**, aaf 5401.

63. Mishima, Y., Honda, C., Ichihashi, M., Obara, H., Hiratsuka, J., Fukuda, H., *et al.* (1989). Treatment of malignant melanoma by single thermal neutron capture therapy with melanoma-seeking ^{10}B-compound. *Lancet* **334**, 388–389.

64. Carpano, M., Perona, M., Rodriguez, C., Nievas, S., Olivera, M., Santa Cruz, G. A., *et al.* (2015). Experimental studies of boronophenylalanine ((10) BPA) biodistribution for the individual application of boron neutron capture therapy (BNCT) for malignant melanoma treatment. *Int. J. Radiat. Oncol. Biol. Phys.* **93**, 344–352.

65. Trivillin, V. A., Garabalino, M. A., Colombo, L. L., González, S. J., Farías, R. O., Monti Hughes, A., *et al.* (2014). Biodistribution of the boron carriers boronophenylalanine (BPA) and/or decahydrodecaborate (GB-10) for boron neutron capture therapy (BNCT) in an experimental model of lung metastases. *Appl. Radiat. Isot.* **88**, 94–98.

66. Suzuki, M., Endo, K., Satoh, H., Sakurai, Y., Kumada, H., Kimura, H., *et al.* (2008). A novel concept of treatment of diffuse or multiple pleural tumors by boron neutron capture therapy (BNCT). *Radiother. Oncol.* **88**, 192–195.

67. Suzuki, M., Sakurai, Y., Masunaga, S., Kinashi, Y., Nagata, K., Maruhashi, A., *et al.* (2007). A preliminary experimental study of boron neutron capture therapy for malignant tumors spreading in thoracic cavity. *Jpn. J. Clin. Oncol.* **37**, 245–249.

68. Suzuki, M., Sakurai, Y., Masunaga, S., Kinashi, Y., Nagata, K., Maruhashi, A., *et al.* (2006). Feasibility of boron neutron capture therapy (BNCT) for malignant pleural mesothelioma from a viewpoint of dose distribution analysis. *Int. J. Radiat. Oncol. Biol. Phys.* **66**, 1584–1589.

69. Berzenji, L. and Van Schil, P. (2018). Multimodality treatment of malignant pleural mesothelioma. *F1000Res.* **7**, 1681.

70. Lagniau, S., Lamote, K., van Meerbeeck, J. P. and Vermaelen, K. Y. (2017). Biomarkers for early diagnosis of malignant mesothelioma: do we need another moonshot? *Oncotarget.* **8**, 53751–53762.

71. Alberti, D., Deagostino, A., Toppino, A., Protti, N., Bortolussi, S., Altieri, S., *et al.* (2018). An innovative therapeutic approach for malignant mesothelioma

treatment based on the use of Gd/boron multimodal probes for MRI guided BNCT. *J. Control. Release* **280**, 31–38.

72. Wang, S., Blaha, C., Santos, R., Huynh, T., Hayes, T. R., Beckford-Vera, D. R., *et al.* (2019). Synthesis and initial biological evaluation of boron-containing prostate-specific membrane antigen ligands for treatment of prostate cancer using boron neutron capture therapy. *Mol. Pharm.* **16**, 3831–3841.

73. Yasui, L., Kroc, T., Gladden, S., Andorf, C., Bux, S. and Hosmane, N. S. (2012). Boron neutron capture in prostate cancer cells. *Appl. Radiat. Isot.* **70**, 6–12.

74. Takagaki, M., Ono, K., Oda, Y., Kikuchi, H., Nemoto, H., Iwamoto, S., *et al.* (1996). Hydroxylforms of p-boronophenylalanine as potential boron carriers on boron neutron capture therapy for malignant brain tumors. *Cancer Res.* **56**, 2017–2020.

75. Pettersson, O. A., Olsson, P., Lindström, P., Sjöberg, S., Larsson, B. S. and Carlsson, J. (1994). Cellular binding of carboranylalanine and some effects of boron neutron capture. analysis of cultured melanoma B16 cells. *Acta Oncol.* **33**, 685–691.

76. Takahara, K., Inamoto, T., Minami, K., Yoshikawa, Y., Takai, T., Ibuki, N., *et al.* (2015). The anti-proliferative effect of boron neutron capture therapy in a prostate cancer xenograft model. *PLoS One* **10**, e0136981.

77. Nedunchezhian, K., Aswath, N., Thiruppathy, M. and Thirugnanamurthy, S. (2016). Boron neutron capture therapy — a literature review. *J. Clin. Diagn. Res.* **10**, ZE01–ZE04.

78. Alkins, R. D., Brodersen, P. M., Sodhi, R. N. S. and Hynynen, K. (2013). Enhancing drug delivery for boron neutron capture therapy of brain tumors with focused ultrasound. *Neuro. Oncol.* **15**, 1225–1235.

79. Sun, T., Li, Y., Huang, Y., Zhang, Z., Yang, W., Du, Z., *et al.* (2016). Targeting glioma stem cells enhances anti-tumor effect of boron neutron capture therapy. *Oncotarget.* **7**, 43095–43108.

80. Barth, R. F., Yang, W., Wu, G., Swindall, M., Byun, Y., Narayanasamy, S., *et al.* (2008). Thymidine kinase 1 as a molecular target for boron neutron capture therapy of brain tumors. *Proc. Natl. Acad. Sci.* **105**, 17493–17497.

81. Zhu, Y., Peng, A. T., Carpenter, K., Maguire, J. A., Hosmane, N. S. and Takagaki, M. (2005). Substituted carborane-appended water-soluble single-wall carbon nanotubes: new approach to boron neutron capture therapy drug delivery. *J. Am. Chem. Soc.* **127**, 9875–9880.

82. Dash, B. P., Satapathy, R., Bode, B. P., Reidl, C. T., Sawicki, J. W., Mason, A. J., *et al.* (2012). "Click" chemistry-mediated phenylene-cored carborane dendrimers. *Organometallics* **31**, 2931–2935.

83. Aryal, M., Arvanitis, C. D., Alexander, P. M. and McDannold, N. (2014). Ultrasound-mediated blood-brain barrier disruption for targeted drug delivery in the central nervous system. *Adv. Drug Deliv. Rev.* **72**, 94–109.

84. Fan, C.-H., Wang, T.-W., Hsieh, Y.-K., Wang, C.-F., Gao, Z., Kim, A., *et al.* (2019). Enhancing boron uptake in brain glioma by a boron-polymer/microbubble

complex with focused ultrasound. *ACS Appl. Mater. Interfaces* **11**, 11144–11156.

85. McCord, E., Pawar, S., Koneru, T., Tatiparti, K., Sau, S. and Iyer, A. K. (2021). Folate receptors' expression in gliomas may possess potential nanoparticle-based drug delivery opportunities. *ACS Omega* **6**, 4111–4118.

85. Shukla, S., Wu, G., Chatterjee, M., Yang, W., Sekido, M., Diop, L. A., *et al.* (2003). Synthesis and biological evaluation of folate receptor-targeted boronated PAMAM dendrimers as potential agents for neutron capture therapy. *Bioconjug. Chem.* **14**, 158–167.

86. Barth, R. F., Mi, P. and Yang, W. (2018). Boron delivery agents for neutron capture therapy of cancer. *Cancer Commun.* **38**, 35.

87. Xiong, H., Zhou, D., Qi, Y., Zhang, Z., Xie, Z., Chen, X., *et al.* (2015). Doxorubicin-loaded carborane-conjugated polymeric nanoparticles as delivery system for combination cancer therapy. *Biomacromolecules* **16**, 3980–3988.

88. Kamaly, N., Yameen, B., Wu, J. and Farokhzad, O. C. (2016). Degradable controlled-release polymers and polymeric nanoparticles: mechanisms of controlling drug release. *Chem. Rev.* **116**, 2602–2663.

89. Huang, M., Deng, J., Gao, L. and Zhou, J. (2020). Innovative strategies to advance CAR T cell therapy for solid tumors. *Am. J. Cancer Res.* **10**, 1979–1992.

90. Mitchell, M. J., Billingsley, M. M., Haley, R. M., Wechsler, M. E., Peppas, N. A. and Langer, R. (2021). Engineering precision nanoparticles for drug delivery. *Nat. Rev. Drug Discov.* **20**, 101–124.

Chapter 4

Application of Theranostic Technology in Boron Neutron Capture Therapy

Yinghuai Zhu,[1,*] Tanzeela Fazal[2]

[1] *Sunshine Lake Pharma Co. Ltd., China*
[2] *Department of Chemistry, Abbottabad University of Science and Technology, Pakistan*

Abstract

Boron neutron capture therapy (BNCT) is a highly targeted, selective and effective technique to cure various types of cancers with reduced harm to the healthy cells. BNCT treatment needs to selectively and homogeneously distribute the ^{10}boron (B) atoms inside the tumor tissues as well as capture sufficient neutrons to initiate a nuclear fission reaction with release of the high linear energy particles to kill the tumor cells. Similar to chemotherapy and other radiotherapies for tumor treatment, theranostics are vital in BNCT. Particularly, *in vivo* localization and quantification of ^{10}B concentrations is critical for the success of BNCT. However, currently both instrumentation and technology do not fulfill accurate measurement and time requirements, so more effectual strategies are desired. This chapter summarizes the currently used diagnostic technologies in BNCT such as magnetic resonance imaging, positron emission tomography, and fluorescence imaging, and discusses emerging imaging techniques as well as boron carriers for BNCT application.

Keywords: boron carriers, boron neutron capture therapy (BNCT), diagnostic imaging, magnetic resonance imaging (MRI), positron emission tomography (PET), fluorescence imaging (FI).

---

*Corresponding author.

4.1 Introduction

4.1.1 *Overview of Boron Neutron Capture Therapy*

For the treatment of cancer, radiation therapy has occupied a prestigious role both in developed and developing countries. It was reported that more than 50% of cancer patients globally need radiotherapy treatments at least once in their course of disease development [1]. In spite of its preponderance, many serious complications are associated with radiotherapy, due to its general non-selectivity and relative ineffectiveness with large and hypoxic tumors, which are particularly damning for patients with recurring cancers. With biological and physical advancements, a number of approaches have been applied to address these issues. Among them, boron neutron capture therapy (BNCT) is a promising technology. BNCT is a binary radiotherapeutic technology based on the boron nuclear fission reaction. In the reaction, an isotope of ^{10}B atom absorbs a neutron to form an ^{11}B atom in an excited state. The ^{11}B atom conducts a nuclear fission reaction to release high linear energy particles, including α (^{4}He), lithium nucleus (^{7}Li) and γ-rays. These particles can cross the membrane and heavily damage the DNA and/or RNA of a tumor cell, thus killing it. A scheme of clinical application of BNCT is shown in Figure 4.1. Since both α (^{4}He) and lithium nucleus (^{7}Li) particles possess a range of less than 10 μm, and that length fits a single cell size (around 10 μm), the BNCT treatment can target the malignant tumor cells while sparing the surrounding normal tissues, achieving precision on a cellular level.

The BNCT concept was first elaborated by Gordon Locher in 1936 [2]. He hypothesized that boron and other elements, which have high thermal neutron capture cross sections, could potentially be applied in therapeutic treatments by virtue of this unique property; in other words, these elements might be selectively and artificially delivered into tissues of the body to be irradiated by thermal neutrons. To verify the above concept, the first radiobiological studies were initiated at the University of Illinois in 1938, and the results of the *in vitro* experiments were reported by Kruger in 1940 [3]. It was found that neoplastic cells can be destroyed by irradiation of thermal neutrons in the presence of boric acid; this implied that if sufficient boron agents were applied to

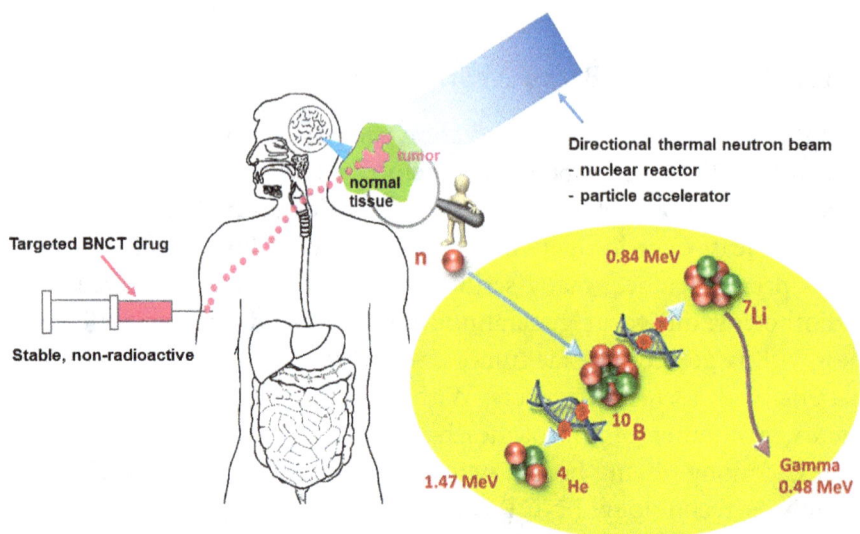

Figure 4.1 A typical scheme of the clinical application of BNCT. The targeted boron drugs are injected and selectively accumulate in tumor parts. After a certain time, the tumor parts in a patient are then irradiated with thermal neutrons. The boron-10 atoms in the BNCT drugs undergo the nuclear fission reactions to release high linear energy particles, which are able to damage and kill the tumor cells.

the tumor *in vivo*, it could be destroyed. In 1951, the first clinical trials of BNCT were conducted by William Herbert Sweet and Gordon Lee Brownell at the Brookhaven Graphite Research Reactor in New York to treat glioblastoma multiforme [4–6]. Unfortunately, all progress in BNCT was halted due to unsuccessful treatment outcomes and toxicities of the boron agents used, which were boric acid and derivatives. Better results were achieved by Sweet *et al.* in 1963, who treated glioma patients *via* BNCT and used *para*-carboxylic phenylboric acid and $Na_2B_{10}H_{10}$ as boron carriers [7]. Decades later, Hatanaka and his colleagues initiated a Japanese BNCT program in 1968 to treat patients with high-grade gliomas using borocaptate sodium (BSH) as boron drug. They reported a median survival of 21.3 months obtained from their clinical results [8]. The stellar outcomes may be driven by the BSH drug because it was found that BSH demonstrated a high tumor-to-normal brain tissue ratio of around 40 to 1 [9,10].

Para-borono-phenylalanine (BPA), which has equal amounts of left-and right-handed enantiomers, was introduced in BNCT by Mishima *et al.* for treating malignant melanomas in the racemic form [11–16]. In the early 1990s, the L enantiomer of BPA was found to be more promising, and commonly used in clinical trials to replace the racemic mixture; thenceforth L-BPA became the most widely used boron carrier in BNCT treatment [12,17]. L-BPA and BSH are regarded as second-generation boron drugs, succeeding the first generation of borax. They are still commonly used in current BNCT treatment. After the 1990s, clinical trials for BNCT were suspended due to a few incidents in various nuclear reactions during the process and research shifted to animal experiments. In 2010, BNCT clinical studies were initiated at the Taipei Veterans General Hospital in Taiwan for patients with previously irradiated and locally recurrent head and neck cancer [18]. A large dose of 500 mg/kg of BPA was used to improve the treatment effects. Between 2013 and 2016, BNCT studies on melanoma patients (22 cases) were carried out at the Third Xiangya Hospital in China with a specialized hospital neutron irradiator and BPA-fructose as the boron carrier [19]. The BPA dose used in the research was 180 mg/kg/h, and exciting results were obtained within 24 months after the BNCT treatment. New neutron sources for BNCT usage are now under construction in mainland China, following the latest development and popularization of neutron sources (see Chapter 5), so BNCT is expected to play more important roles in cancer treatment in China.

On the other hand, it is well recognized that the success of radiotherapy is highly dependent on the precise definition of the tumor lesions, rational treatment plan and accurate delivery of the radiation dose to the tumor tissue. Medical imaging enables a medical professional to recreate images of various parts of the body for diagnostic or treatment purposes, and is a central part of the improved outcomes of modern medicine. Imaging techniques have been widely used in diagnosing, staging, treatment simulation, treatment planning, treatment delivery, localization and response assessment. The advances in imaging technology have increased accuracy in treatment delivery and improved the applications of new techniques in radiotherapy. As a result, treatment-related toxicities in radiation oncology have been reduced and tumor control rates improved for cancer patients.

4.1.2 Brief Survey of Medical Imaging

In the course of development of medical imaging, X-ray imaging was the earliest form, which was first demonstrated by Roentgen in 1895 [20]. Later, computed tomography (CT), also known as computerized axial tomography, emerged and replaced X-rays [21]. CT imaging uses specialized X-ray equipment and provides cross-sectional images, as shown in Figure 4.2. CT is a non-invasive medical examination which has been used for various diagnostic and therapeutic purposes.

Magnetic resonance imaging (MRI) emerged at the end of the 20th century, and is a medical application of nuclear magnetic resonance (NMR). Superconducting magnets and radio waves are utilized to create a strong magnetic field and generate images of organs and tissues. MRI helps doctors examine a patient's soft tissues and organs and diagnose tumors. The first clinical magnetic resonance images were created in 1980 [22,23]. Although MRI had showed limited diagnostic application in the beginning, it was improved significantly in practice, and has become a widely available, powerful clinical imaging modality. MRI has been used for cancer detection, diagnosis, and treatment monitoring and assessment.

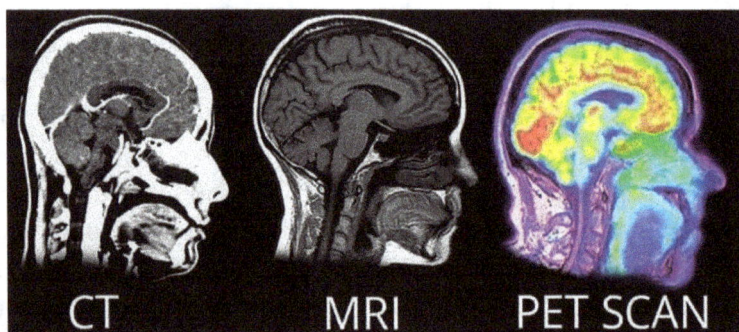

Figure 4.2 Representative scanning images of the head by CT, MRI and PET [28].

Positron emission tomography (PET) is also an important advanced medical imaging technique used in clinical settings (Figure 4.2) [24]. In principle, PET is a radiopharmaceutical scintillography technique used in nuclear medicine. The radioactive isotopes are attached to certain molecules to form so-called labelled molecules or radiotracers, such as glucose and drugs, and are injected into the body to be taken up by certain tissues. In the tissues, the radiotracer undergoes a beta plus decay and emits a positron [25]. The releasing positron collides with an electron and emits gamma rays which can be detected by gamma cameras to form a three-dimensional image [25]. PET imaging has been combined with CT imaging, known as PET-CT scanning, to help in further narrowing down a diagnosis. PET imaging allows *in vivo* tracing of a chemical in the biological pathway. Thus far, ^{18}F isotope is one of the commonly used radionuclides, and the carbohydrate derivative fluorodeoxyglucose (^{18}F-FDG) is the most commonly used radiotracer [26].

Fluorescence imaging (FI) is another useful tool in hospitals to diagnose and monitor diseases such as infectious and non-communicable diseases [27]. It is a cost-effective imaging modality, and is helpful to study complex samples which cannot be thoroughly investigated by regular microscopy. The imaging technique has been well developed recently, and less expensive fluorescence microscopes are commercially available, which may further support diagnostic research in laboratories. Nevertheless, the light and antibody/dye penetration may be significantly hampered by the tissues, so further advances in knowledge and equipment are necessary for real-life application.

It has been noted that diagnostic methods, pre-treatment simulation and a well-constructed treatment plan (this Chapter) play irreplaceable roles in BNCT treatment besides a feasible boron agent (Chapter 3) and high-quality neutron source (Chapter 5). Before subjecting to neutron irradiation, precise and accurate evaluation of both tumor location and concentration of ^{10}B in different tissues of a patient is obligatory to plot a rational and effective BNCT clinical treatment regime [29,30]. The following methods are commonly used to evaluate the ^{10}B concentrations within targeted tissues in a patient.

(1) After injection of the boron drug, blood or tissue samples of the patient are taken after a certain time and subjected to *ex vivo* analysis of the ^{10}B concentration, which are extrapolated according to the pharmacokinetic and pharmacodynamic parameters of the drug. The conventional instrumentation and methods to analyze ^{10}B concentration in biological samples include inductively coupled plasma mass spectrometer (ICP-MS), inductively coupled plasma atomic emission spectroscopy (ICP-AES), high-performance liquid chromatography mass spectroscopy (HPLC-MS), and prompt gamma-ray analysis (PGRA). The inherent drawback of the strategy is that it is impossible to gain accurate information on the ^{10}B concentration and distribution in an individual patient due to the heterogeneity of tumor tissues.

(2) After injection of the boron drug, the targeted tissues or organs of the patient are subjected to imaging estimation and evaluation after a certain time to provide information on the ^{10}B concentration and distribution. Currently, the image fusion techniques of PET and CT are widely used in many BNCT facilities. The fusion technique allows the merging of two or more imaging datasets into a single file, and thus combines the advantages of PET imaging and CT scan. PET imaging aims to identify and localize the tumor tissues, whereas CT provides important information on the anatomical details of the studied lesions [25–27].

In the future of BNCT treatment, body imaging techniques, which enable *in vivo* assessment of the ^{10}B concentration and distribution in a lesion, will play more important roles because the rational treatment plans are mainly based on the information obtained thereby. This might be the final push required for BNCT to be practically successful, even though it remains challenging at present due to limited accessibility of advanced diagnostic facilities in many underdeveloped countries. This chapter summarizes the current clinical applications of advanced imaging techniques such as MRI and PET in BNCT, and discusses the importance of incorporating concurrent imaging to achieve a precise and effective BNCT treatment.

4.2. Magnetic Resonance Imaging in BNCT

In BNCT treatment, MRI can be used to detect tumors or cancer in a patient's brain, liver, breast, and other organs. It helps doctors to analyze the tumor anatomy to gain information on the tumor location and size before and after BNCT. Theoretically, the current clinically used boron drugs, BPA and BSH, can also be analyzed by MRI based on boron NMR [31–34]. However, translation of the NMR spectroscopy of boron into clinical application for human subjects requires special hardware and software to provide strong magnetic fields and generate images of organs and tissues. The facilities are not available so far, and are an area for further development. In future, the following issues should be addressed for MRI application in BNCT to non-invasively examine the boron concentration and biodistribution.

(1) Elemental boron has two naturally occurring and stable isotopes, ^{10}B and ^{11}B, with the natural abundance of 19.65% and 80.35%, respectively. The two boron isotopes both show magnetic activity, and can be determined by NMR spectroscopy. However, ^{10}B nucleus has a low sensitivity of 0.396% relative to ^{1}H at natural abundance, a low gyromanetic ratio of 4.6 MHz/T, and a high quadrupole moment [35]. All these make it difficult to analyze ^{10}B *in vivo* using MRI.

(2) On the other hand, ^{11}B nucleus has a high sensitivity of 16.5% relative to ^{1}H at natural abundance; most of the boron NMR spectroscopy carried out in chemistry research deals with ^{11}B. Nevertheless, ^{10}B-enriched (>95%) boron drugs are commonly used to improve the BNCT effect, and as a result the concentration of ^{11}B is low, which weakens its MRI signal. In addition, the ^{11}B nucleus has a spin quantum number of 3/2, and the relaxation time (T2) is short, which may cause a total decay of the signal before imaging. Therefore, special methods are required to create ^{11}B NMR images [35–37].

In 1988, the first ^{11}B image of a BNCT agent was reported, where a back-projection technique was employed [36]. The sodium salt,

$Na_4B_{24}H_{22}S_2$, a dimer of BSH, was prepared and used as the boron drug at a dose of 250 µg of boron per gram of body weight in the work. It was suggested that sensitivity enhancement was required before ^{11}B imaging could be clinically useful. Soon after, the same group reported *in vivo* distribution and pharmacokinetics of the same BNCT agent non-invasively in 1991 [37]. The results further demonstrate the capability of MRI to non-invasively monitor the distribution and excretion of boron agents *in vivo*.

MRI technology was also used to detect the pharmaceutical properties of current clinically used BPA. In principle, the signal of ^{10}B magnetic resonance could be used to create the images of the ^{10}B-enriched BPA *in vivo*. However, the transverse relaxation time (T2) of ^{10}B nucleus in BPA is too short due to the electronic cloud asymmetry at the quadrupolar nucleus site [38], and consequently the resulting ^{10}B images show a low resolution which is inadequate for BNCT application. Thus the ^{10}B-based MRI technique is not suitable to determine BPA. The ^1H-based MRI technique is not applicable to map BPA either because of the intense ^1H background signal *in vivo*, which are derived from all the surrounding tissues and bloods composed of various organic and inorganic molecules. The ^1H signals of the boron drugs are therefore too weak to be used in clinics. The application of ^1H-based MRI in BNCT was reported for two patients in 1999 to investigate the BPA-fructose complex in their brain tissues *in vivo* [39]. The protons in the benzene ring of the BPA molecule were set as a NMR signature to identify and measure BPA *in vivo*. Soon after, ^1H-based magnetic resonance spectroscopy (MRS) and magnetic resonance spectroscopy imaging (MRSI) were used to detect BPA in animal tests *in vivo* [40]. MRS and MRSI are non-invasive techniques based on the same physical principles as MRI and can be used to measure the concentrations of different chemical components within tissues [41].

On the other hand, the ^{18}F-labeled L-4-borono-2-fluorophenylalanine (^{18}F-BPA) has been introduced in BNCT and used as a radiotracer to perform PET imaging in clinics [42, 43]. This imaging method can gain information on the *in vivo* spatial distribution of ^{10}B. However, it does not provide helpful chemical-pharmacological information on the boron drugs due to the relatively low image resolution. Furthermore, application of the radioactive ^{18}F nuclide constrains the time in drug synthesis and clinical administration due to its limited half-life (~110 minutes). Therefore, ^{19}F-based MRI methods have been studied to detect *in vivo* spatial distribution of the non-radioactive L-4-borono-2-fluorophenylalanine (^{19}F-BPA) [44–46]. ^{19}F-MRI and ^{19}F-MRS have been reported to provide useful information on ^{19}F-BPA pharmaceutics on small rodents. It was confirmed that the maximum uptake of ^{19}F-BPA-fructose complex within the tumor was at 2.5 h after infusion in C6 glioma-bearing rats [46]. The results suggest that ^{19}F-MRI and ^{19}F-MRS could potentially be used in BNCT clinics to map and detect the distribution of boron drugs *in vivo*, as well as to follow the pharmacokinetics and pharmacodynamics of the drugs. In addition, the clinically used MRI scanners can be used to perform ^{19}F-MRI after minor improvements and suitable tuning radiofrequency coils.

In MRI, the image quality of internal body structures can be improved by using an MRI contrast agent, which may shorten the relaxation times of nuclei within body tissues. Gadolinium-based compounds, such as gadopentetic acid (Gd-DTPA) and gadoteric acid (Gd-DOTA), are commonly used as contrast agents for MRI enhancement [47]. Therefore, a boron drug can be attached to the gadolinium compound to improve the MRI imaging concerned with *in vivo* boron quantitation. Both Gd-DTPA and Gd-DOTA have been functionalized with a carborane and BPA species, respectively, as shown in Figure 4.3 [48–50]. Nevertheless, the modification of the molecular structure of BPA significantly decreases its tumor tendency *in vivo*, and makes it unsuitable for BNCT application. Therefore, nanoscale drug carriers such as low-density lipoproteins have been employed to selectively deliver the above mentioned complexes to target tumor tissues [51]. It should be noted that naturally occurring gadolinium-157 (^{157}Gd) has a neutron capture cross section of 254,000 barns, which is around 66 times higher with respect to that of ^{10}B. ^{157}Gd is thus potentially useful as a neutron-absorbing isotope for neutron capture therapy (NCT). Indeed, GdNCT is considered as a promising cancer treatment option, and more developments are underway [52].

Functional nanomaterials can be rationally designed to overcome limitations of free therapeutics and navigate biological barriers such as

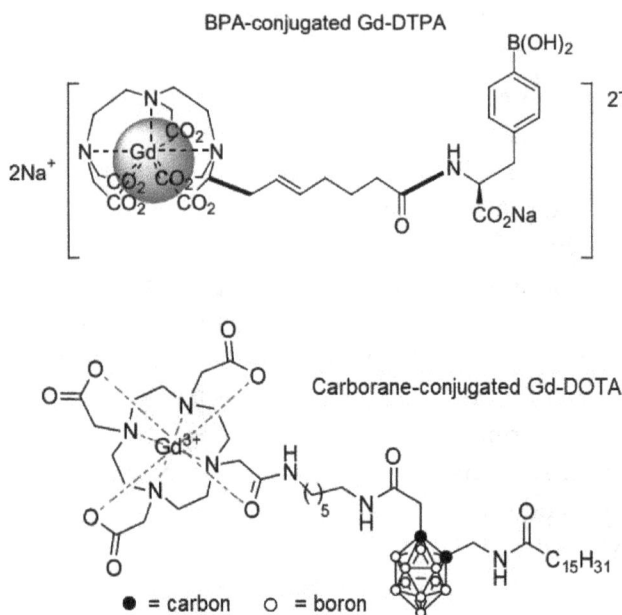

Figure 4.3 Molecular structures of BPA-Gd-DTPA and Carborane-Gd-DOTA.

the blood-brain barrier (BBB), and thus significantly improve diagnosis and treatment specificity [53]. Therefore, boron-engineered nanomaterials hold significant promise to enhance the BNCT treatment. Applications in BNCT of nanocomposites containing boron, gadolinium and iron were studied in pre-clinical investigations [54–58]. A nanocomposite made of folic acid and $GdBO_3$-Fe_3O_4 was constructed and investigated *in vitro* as a next-generation boron agent for magnetically targeted therapy, FI, MRI diagnosis and NCT [55]. In 2015, a dual boron/Gd compound made of low-density lipoprotein (LDL) carrier and carborane-Gd-DOTA (shown in Figure 4.3) was reported as an innovative theranostic agent [56]. It was able to maximize the selective uptake of boron atoms in tumor cells and quantitatively detect the *in vivo* boron distribution by MRI. The nanomaterial was found to target LDL receptors, which are overexpressed on various tumor cells [56,57]. It was described to enhance BNCT with promising reduction of malignant mesothelioma with respect to the control group [57]. Kuthala *et al.* reported a ^{10}B-enriched boron nanoparticle, whose surface was functionalized by fluorescein isothiocyanate, Gd(III)-DTPA complex and RGD-K peptides [58]. The nanomaterial was claimed to be able to cross the BBB, and selectively target glioblastoma multiforme brain tumors. A high delivery dose of 50.5 µg ^{10}B/g tumor cells was achieved with a tumor-to-blood boron ratio of 2.8. It is apparent that nanoparticles can enhance the contrast of the MRI, help diagnose the brain tumor and guide the BNCT treatment to prolong the half-life of animal models [58].

4.3 Positron Emission Tomography/Computed Tomography Scanning in BNCT

PET produces three-dimensional scanned maps, and is one of the most useful methods in clinics to gain information on *in vivo* biochemical and pharmacological processes. Advanced developments have been made in PET techniques to improve image quality while reducing the detection time. PET-CT scanning has been introduced in BNCT to examine the spatial distribution of ^{10}B in associated tissues [59–61]. In 1991, Ishiwata *et al.* reported the synthesis and potential application of ^{18}F-BPA in BNCT [59]. The racemic compound was prepared by direct fluorination of BPA as shown in Scheme 4.1, followed by HPLC purification, in radiochemical yields of 25–35% and with a radiochemical purity of over 99%. The racemic ^{18}F-BPA was found to be a potentially effective radiotracer for PET imaging. Soon after, the same research group studied the *in vivo* uptake by PET using pure L-[^{18}F]-FBPA enantiomer in animal models [60]. The results suggested that L-[^{18}F]-FBPA could be used as a probe for BPA in BNCT treatment of malignant melanomas to localize the tumor lesion and determine the ^{10}B

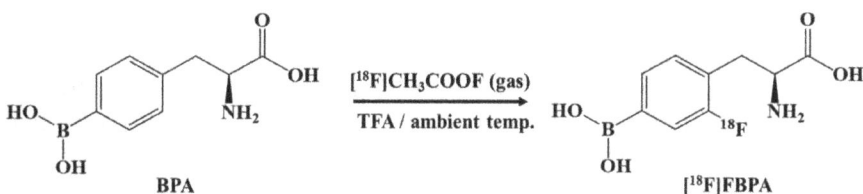

Scheme 4.1 Synthesis of ^{18}F-FBPA.

concentration in tissues. A ^{10}B-based single-photon emission computed tomography (SPECT) was also investigated to measure the ^{10}B concentration in tumor cells [61]. The technique can create an online three-dimensional image, and when combined with PGRA, can provide accurate dose estimation for BNCT. Nevertheless, the technique can only determine boron concentration during the administration of BNCT treatment, and thus makes it challenging to formulate a rational treatment plan.

In 2013, Ishiwata et al. studied dynamic whole-body PET scanning in humans using L-[^{18}F]-FBPA as a radiotracer [62]. It was found that the radiation dosimetry of the L-[^{18}F]-FBPA presented an effective dose of 23.9 µSv/MBq (n = 6) in humans, which was similar to other ^{18}F-fluorinated PET tracers such as 6-^{18}F-fluorol-dopa (19.9 µSv/MBq) and ^{18}F-FDG (19–29 µSv/MBq). It was also claimed that estimated effective doses from the mouse-derived data were inconsistent with that of the human-derived data due to interspecies differences in pharmacokinetics between human subjects and mice and differences in the methodology of biodistribution measurements. Therefore, whole-body imaging for the investigation of radiation dosimetry is strongly recommended as an initial clinical trial when evaluating a new PET tracer. Later, Kono et al. reported a smaller effective dose of ^{18}F-FBPA compared with ^{18}F-FDG in adult (3 men, 3 women; age range, 28–68 years) and pediatric patients (3 patients; age range, 5–12 years) [63]. Adult patients had significantly smaller absorbed doses than pediatric patients. The effective dose of ^{18}F-FBPA in pediatric patients (31 µSv/MBq, n = 3) was larger than that in adult patients (15 µSv/MBq, n = 6). The mean effective dose was 57% lower in adult patients compared with pediatric patients.

In BNCT treatment, the ^{10}B concentration in the blood is commonly used as the reference to evaluate the ^{10}B concentration in tumors [64]. Therefore, in a practical clinical treatment, the ^{10}B concentration in tumors is calculated by multiplying the ^{10}B concentration in the blood by the tumor-to-blood ratio. Both the ^{10}B concentration in the blood and the ratio are measured by ^{18}F-FBPA PET during neutron irradiation [65]. However, estimation of the ^{10}B concentration in the surrounding normal tissues by ^{18}F-FBPA PET did not present reasonable accuracy compared to that of the ^{10}B concentration in blood. The PET method thus cannot be used to predict possible adverse effects on the normal tissues by neutron irradiation in BNCT. And as a result, pharmacokinetic analysis continues to be used to calculate the *in vivo* ^{10}B concentrations.

Nowadays, the ^{18}F-FBPA PET has been utilized in BNCT for patients with different types of tumors such as malignant brain tumors [66–68], recurrent head and neck cancers [69,70], and malignant melanomas [71] in many clinical studies. ^{18}F-FBPA PET has been a part of the inclusion criteria for BNCT clinical phase trials to accurately detect tumor lesions which are challenging to determine by other technologies such as MRI. In Finnish and Taiwanese studies, ^{18}F-FBPA PET was performed both before and after BNCT to evaluate treatment response in recurrent head and neck cancers [72–76]. In 2022, a carefully planned two fractions of salvage BNCT strategy with low dosage each time was performed in Taiwan to treat life-threatening patients with end-stage brainstem glioma [77]. The ^{10}B-4-borono-L-phenylalanine (L-BPA) was administrated as the boron drug, and ^{18}F-BPA-PET was used to estimate boron concentration as shown in Figure 4.4. It was reported that the two fractionated low-dose BNCT did not cause acute

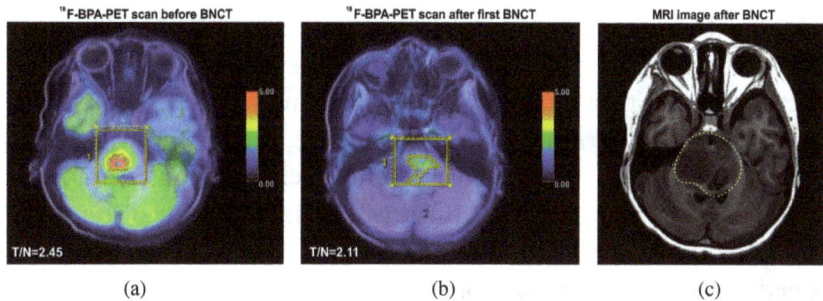

Figure 4.4 The ^{18}F-BPA-PET and MRI images of a patient with brainstem glioma. (a) The ^{18}F-BPA-PET reveals the location of tumor activity before BNCT treatment. (b) The ^{18}F-BPA-PET reveals the location of tumor with reduced tumor activity after first procedure of BNCT treatment. (c) The follow-up MRI image of the patient shows radiation necrosis in the fourth ventricle (dashed yellow line). The yellow squares indicate the tumor location before and after BNCT treatment [77].

or late adverse effects on the patients with end-stage brainstem tumors. Moreover, ^{18}F-FDG PET was reported to help evaluate maxillary sinus cancer post-BNCT radiotherapy [78].

In summary, ^{18}F-FBPA PET helps quantitatively and non-invasively evaluate the ^{10}B concentrations in human blood and tissues to grant a successful BNCT clinical treatment. It has also been used to assess the curative effect and prognosis of patients after BNCT treatment. However, the half-life of ^{18}F is relatively short (~108 min), so it remains a big challenge to complete the labeling, transportation, and injection of the ^{18}F-FBPA drug in such a limited time. Therefore, radioisotopes other than ^{18}F have been incorporated to boron-containing compounds in studies. Gold nanoparticles were reported to be labeled with iodine ^{123}I [79] or ^{124}I [80] for mice investigations. ^{64}Cu was also explored as an alternative [81,82]. It was claimed that a BSH derivative fused with a short arginine peptide (1R, 2R, 3R) and labeled with ^{64}Cu showed a high uptake by brain tumors [82]. Other radioactive nuclides-based PET imaging, such as ^{177}Lu PET, could also be studied as candidates to replace ^{18}F-FBPA PET [83].

4.4 Fluorescence Imaging in BNCT

Currently, non-invasive FI is widely used in biological imaging due to its high selectivity, high sensitivity and diversity [27]. As abovementioned, FI requires a fluorescent probe and a suitable light source. The light excites the probe to produce fluorescence signals for biological imaging, both *in vitro* and *in vivo*. Therefore, the functionalized fluorescent probes play important roles to effectively distinguish tumor cells (or tissues) from normal cells (or tissues), facilitating early diagnosis. FI is thus a sensitive spectroscopic technique that can be potentially applied for the estimation of boron distribution among the various partitions of the tissues.

Various fluorophores, such as dipyrromethene, porphyrin and phtalocianine, have been investigated in pre-clinical BNCT research. Kalot *et al.* incorporated the clinically used ^{10}B-BSH with a water-soluble aza-boron-dipyrromethene dyes (BODIPY) fluorophore to enhance the ^{10}B-BSH tumor vectorization [84]. The fluorescent aza-BODIPY/^{10}B-BSH compound was reported to be able to image ^{10}B-BSH in the tumor area. Recently, it was reported that the terminal zwitterions of BODIPY polymers could tightly wrap boron clusters such as carborane ($C_2B_{10}H_{12}$) and decaborane ($B_{10}H_{14}$) to form small corresponding nanoclusters [85]. The borane polymers were found to be highly selective in accumulating in the subcutaneous tumor sites of mice over time based on the *in vivo* FI. In addition, BODIPY-based phosphors are sufficiently hydrophobic, so they can easily cross the lipid layers of cell membranes and bind with hydrophobic fragments of proteins. At present, BODIPY-based dyes are under active investigation for staining the cores of cellular organelles and labelling individual biomolecules [86]. The boronated BODIPYs are thus potential fluorescent markers and warrant further study for BNCT applications.

Porphyrins have been extensively studied as potential photosensitizers in photodynamic therapy [87–89]. Smilowitz *et al.* employed the newer, non-toxic lipophilic porphyrins, 5,10,15,20-tetrakis-(3-[1,2-dicarba-closo-dodecaboranyl]methoxyphenyl)-porphyrin ligand-coordinated copper (II) and zinc (II) complexes for FI in tissues of tumor-bearing mice [90]. It was reported that the Zn (II) complex showed fluorescence from liver, spleen and tumor tissues. Furthermore, such fluorescence in the tumors was cytoplasmic but, unlike liver fluorescence, was macroscopically heterogeneous [90]. To develop an efficient quantitative imaging technique to localize and accurately analyze boron concentration for BNCT, a boronated porphyrin nanocomplex (BPN) comprised of the boronated porphyrin and a biocompatible poly(lactide-co-glycolide)-monomethoxy-poly(polyethylene-glycol) (PLGA-mPEG) micelle was studied as a potential theranostic boron agent [91]. The species was found to coordinate with ^{64}Cu(II) to perform PET imaging. According to the FI and PET images, the BPN gave extraordinarily high ratios of tumor to normal tissues; ratios of tumors to liver, muscle, fat, and blood were 3.24 ± 0.22, 61.46 ± 20.26, 31.55 ± 10.30, and 33.85 ± 5.73, respectively. The *in vivo* BNCT using BPN as boron delivery agent completely suppressed tumor growth in mice [91]. It was also observed that porphyrins and phthalocyanines show improved uptake and good persistence in tissues. This unique property may benefit boron delivery for BNCT.

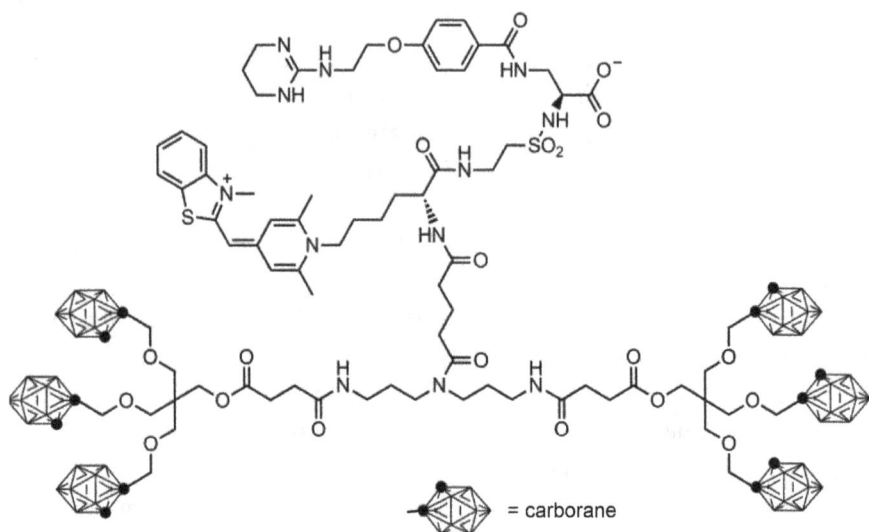

Figure 4.5 Structure of the trifunctional theranostic agent designed by Dubey *et al.* [93].

A disadvantage of porphyrins and phthalocyanines is their limited solubility in aqueous media and common organic solvents. Polyhedral boron derivatives of porphyrins and phthalocyanines are currently under active investigation due to the high boron concentrations of the boron clusters [92].

A new trifunctional theranostic agent was designed for BNCT application by Dubey *et al.* in 2015 [93]. The agent (shown in Figure 4.5) contains a dendritic wedge with high boron content for BNCT and boron MRI, a monomethine cyanine dye as fluorescent marker for FI, and an integrin ligand for efficient tumor targeting selectivity towards the $\alpha_v\beta_3$ receptors. It was reported that the trifunctional agent rapidly and specifically accumulated in the solid tumors in murine subcutaneous tumor xenografts according to the live animal FI images and *ex vivo* analysis of the compound biodistribution. This macromolecular theranostic agent can be used for targeted delivery of a high boron load into solid tumors for future applications in BNCT.

4.5 Summary and Outlook

For a successful BCNT, a boron concentration of 20~50 μg of ^{10}B per gram of tumor tissues is necessary, with tumor-to-normal tissues and tumor-to-blood ratios greater than three. Consequently, the *in vivo* localization and quantification of ^{10}B-containing drugs is mandatory. The failure to do so accurately restricts the successful clinical application of BNCT. Currently, the ^{10}B concentration in the blood is analyzed through estimated boron concentration after injecting the boron carrier into the human body for a certain time, but this method is far from exact. It cannot provide the precise dynamic information on the biodistribution and pharmacokinetics of the boron drugs, as well as the ratio of boron concentration in each site of the tumor to the normal tissues and blood, and thus is unable to completely solve the real-time problem of estimating the radiation dose for BNCT application. The latest developments in MRI, PET and FI are encouraging, though these methods retain disadvantages and limitations. Nowadays, PET (PET-CT) is used in clinics to evaluate the boron concentrations in various tissues and help design a scientific BNCT treatment plan. Dose tracking and evaluation based on MRI has attracted growing attention, and the synthesis of new types of boron theranostics has taken on greater urgency. The combination of clinical imaging and conventional analysis methods such as ICP-MS and FT-IR should be more effective than a singular approach.

References

1. Rosenblatt, E. and Zubizarreta, E. (2017). *Radiotherapy in Cancer Care: Facing the Global Challenge*. International Atomic Energy Agency, p. 5.
2. Locher, G. L. (1936). Biological effects and therapeutic possibilities of neutrons. *Am. J. Roentgenol. Radium. Ther.* **36**, 1–13.
3. Kruger, P. G. (1940). Some biological effects of nuclear disintegration products on neoplastic tissue. *Proc. Natl. Acad. Sci.* **26**, 181–192.
4. Farr, L. E., Sweet, W. H. and Locksley, H. B. (1954). Neutron capture therapy of gliomas using boron. *Trans. Am. Neurol. Assoc.* **13**, 110–113.
5. Farr, L. E., Sweet, W. H., Robertson, J. S., Foster, C. G., Locksley, H. B., Sutherland, D. L., *et al.* (1954). Neutron capture therapy with boron in the

treatment of glioblastoma multiforme. *Am. J. Roentgenol Radium. Ther. Nucl. Med.* **71**, 279–293.

6. Goodwin, J. T., Farr, L. E., Sweet, W. H. and Robertson, J. S. (1955). Pathological study of eight patients with glioblastoma multiforme treated by neutron-capture therapy using boron 10. *Cancer* **8**, 601–615.

7. Brownell, G. L., Murray, B. W., Sweet, W. H., Wellum, G. R. and Soloway, A. H. (1972). A reassessment of neutron capture therapy in the treatment of cerebral gliomas. *Proc. Natl. Cancer Conf.* **7**, 827–837.

8. Hatanaka, H. (1990). Clinical results of boron neutron capture therapy. *Basic Life Sci.* **54**, 15–21.

9. Verbakel, W. F., Sauerwein, W. and Hideghety, K. (2003). Boron concentrations in brain during boron neutron capture therapy: in vivo measurements from the phase I trial EORTC 11961 using a gamma-ray telescope. *Int. J. Radiat. Oncol. Biol. Phys.* **55**, 743–756.

10. Hideghety, K., Sauerwein, W., Wittig, A., Gotz, C., Paquis, P., Grochulla, F., *et al.* (2003). Tissue uptake of BSH in patients with glioblastoma in the EORTC 11961 phase I BNCT trial. *J. Neurooncol.* **62**, 145–156.

11. Ishiwata, K., Ido, T., Kawamura, M., Kubota, K., Ichihashi, M. and Mishima, Y. (1991). 4-Borono-2-[^{18}F]fluoro-D,L-phenylalanine as a target compound for boron neutron capture therapy: tumor imaging potential with positron emission tomography. *Int. J. Rad. Appl. Instrum. B.* **18**, 745–751.

12. Ishiwata, K., Ido, T., Mejia, A. A., Ichihashi, M. and Mishima, Y. (1991). Synthesis and radiation dosimetry of 4-borono-2-[^{18}F]fluoro-D,L-phenylalanine: a target compound for PET and boron neutron capture therapy. *Int. J. Rad. Appl. Instrum. A.* **42**, 325–328.

13. Ishiwata, K., Shiono, M., Kubota, K., Yoshino, K., Hatazawa, J., Ido, T., *et al.* (1992). A unique in vivo assessment of 4-[^{10}B]borono-L-phenylalanine in tumor tissues for boron neutron capture therapy of malignant melanomas using positron emission tomography and 4-borono-2-[^{18}F]fluoro-L-phenylalanine. *Melanoma Res.* **2**, 171–179.

14. Mishima, Y., Honda, C., Ichihashi, M., Obara, H., Hiratsuka, J., Fukuda, H., *et al.* (1989). Treatment of malignant melanoma by single thermal neutron capture therapy with melanoma-seeking ^{10}B-compound. *Lancet* **2**, 388–389.

15. Yoshino, K., Kajiyama, Y., Honda, T., Mori, Y., Honda, C., Ichihashi, M. and Mishima, Y. (1989). A trial to improve the analysis of boron in biological materials. *Pigment Cell Res.* **2**, 286–290.

16. Yoshino, K., Suzuki, A., Mori, Y., Kakihana, H., Honda, C., Mishima, Y., *et al.* (1989). Improvement of solubility of p-boronophenylalanine by complex formation with monosaccharides. *Strahlenther Onkol.* **165**, 127–129.

17. Coderre, J. A., Glass, J. D., Fairchild, R. G., Micca, P. L., Fand, I. and Joel, D. D. (1990). Selective delivery of boron by the melanin precursor analogue

p-boronophenylalanine to tumors other than melanoma. *Cancer Res.* **50**, 138–141.

18. https://clinicaltrials.gov/ct2/show/NCT01173172.
19. Yong, Z., Song, Z., Zhou, Y., Liu, T., Zhang, Z., Zhao, Y., *et al.* (2016). Boron neutron capture therapy for malignant melanoma: first clinical case report in China. *Chin. J. Cancer Res.* **28**, 634–640.
20. Kevles, B. H. (1996). *Naked to the Bone: Medical Imaging in the Twentieth Century.* Rutgers University Press, pp. 19–22.
21. Seeram, E. (2018). Computed tomography: a technical review. *Radiol. Technol.* **89**, 279CT-302CT.
22. Hawkes, R. C., Holland, G. N., Moore, W. S. and Worthington, B. S. (1980). Nuclear magnetic resonance (NMR) tomography of the brain: a preliminary clinical assessment with demonstration of pathology. *J. Comput. Assist. Tomogr.* **4**, 577–586.
23. Smith, F. W., Hutchison, J. M., Mallard, J. R., Johnson, G., Redpath, T. W., Selbie, R. D. *et al.* (1981). Oesophageal carcinoma demonstrated by whole-body nuclear magnetic resonance imaging. *Br. Med. J. (Clin. Res. Ed.)* **282**, 510–512.
24. Bailey, D. L., Townsend, D. W., Valk, P. E. and Maisy, M. N. (2005). *Positron Emission Tomography: Basic Sciences.* Springer.
25. http://hyperphysics.phy-astr.gsu.edu/hbase/Nuclear/nucmed.html#c1.
26. Almuhaideb, A., Papathanasiou, N. and Bomanji, J. (2011). ^{18}F-FDG PET/CT imaging in oncology. *Ann. Saudi. Med.* **31**(1), 3–13.
27. https://sdbif.org/whats-the-difference-between-all-the-different-head-scans.
28. https://apps.who.int/iris/handle/10665/119734.
29. Hosmane, N. S., Maguire, J. A., Zhu, Y. and Takagaki, M. (Eds.) (2012). *Boron and Gadolinium Neutron Capture Therapy for Cancer Treatment.* World Scientific.
30. Skwierawska, D., López-Valverde, J. A., Balcerzyk, M. and Leal, A. (2022). Clinical viability of boron neutron capture therapy for personalized radiation treatment. *Cancers* **14**, 2865.
31. Bendel, P. (2012). Boron Imaging: Localized Quantitative Detection and Imaging of Boron by Magnetic Resonance. In: Sauerwein, W. A. G., Wittig, A., Moss, R. and Nakagawa, Y. (Eds.), *Neutron Capture Therapy: Principles and Applications,* Springer, pp. 2113–2223.
32. Bendel, P., Frantz, A., Zilberstein, J., Kabalka, G. W. and Salomon, Y. (1998). Boron-11 NMR of borocaptate: Relaxation and in vivo detection in melanoma-bearing mice. *Magn. Reson. Med.* **39**, 439–447.
33. Bendel, P. and Sauerwein, W. (2001). Optimal detection of the neutron capture therapy agent borocaptate sodium (BSH): A comparison between H-1 and B-10 NMR. *Med. Phys.* **28**, 178–183.
34. Bendel, P., Wittig, A., Basilico, F., Mauri, P. L. and Sauerwein, W. (2010). Metabolism of borono-phenylalanine-fructose complex (BPA-fr) and borocaptate

sodium (BSH) in cancer patients-results from EORTC trial 11001. *J. Pharm. Biomed. Anal.* **51**, 284–287.

35. Nöth, H. and Wrackmeyer, B. (1978). Nuclear Magnetic Properties of Boron. In: Nöth, H. and Wrackmeyer, B. (Eds.), *Nuclear Magnetic Resonance Spectroscopy of Boron Compounds*, Springer, pp. 5–14.

36. Kabalka, G. W., Davis, M. and Bendel, P. (1988). Boron-11 MRI and MRS of intact animals infused with a boron neutron capture agent. *Magn. Reson. Med.* **8**, 231–237.

37. Kabalka, G. W., Cheng, G. Q., Bendel, P., Micca, P. L. and Slatkin, D. N. (1991). In vivo boron-11 MRI and MRS using $(B_{24}H_{22}S_2)^{4-}$ in the rat. *Magn Reson Imaging.* **9**, 969–973.

38. Abragam, A. (1982). *Principles of Nuclear Magnetism*. Claredon Press.

39. Zuo, C. S., Prasad, P. V., Busse, P., Tang, L. and Zamenhof, R. G. (1999). Proton nuclear magnetic resonance measurement of pboronophenylalanine (BPA): A therapeutic agent for boron neutron capture therapy. *Med. Phys.* **26**, 1230–1236.

40. Bendel, P., Margalit, R. and Salomon, Y. (2005). Optimized 1H MRS and MRSI methods for the in vivo detection of boronophenylalanine. *Magn. Reson. Med.* **53**, 1166–1171.

41. Glunde, K., Jiang, L., Moestue, S. A. and Gribbestad, I. S. (2011). MRS and MRSI guidance in molecular medicine: targeting and monitoring of choline and glucose metabolism in cancer. *NMR Biomed.* **24**, 673–690.

42. Imahori, Y., Ueda, S., Ohmori, Y., Kusuki, T., Ono, K., Fujii, R., *et al.* (1998). Fluorine-18-labeled fluoroboronophenylalanine PET in patients with glioma. *J. Nucl. Med.* **39**, 325–333.

43. Wang, H. L., Liao, A. H., Deng, W. P., Chang, P. F., Chen, J. C., Chen, F. D., *et al.* (2004). Evaluation of 4-borono-2-^{18}F-fluoro-L-phenylalanine-fructose as a probe for boron neutron capture therapy in a glioma-bearing rat model. *J. Neurooncol.* **45**, 302–308.

44. Porcari, P., Capuani, S., Campanella, R., Bella, A. L., Migneco, L. M. and Maraviglia, B. (2006). Biology, Multi-nuclear MRS and ^{19}F MRI of ^{19}F-labelled and [10]B-enriched p-boronophenylalaninefructose complex to optimize boron neutron capture therapy: phantom studies at high magnetic fields. *Phys. Med. Biol.* **51**, 3141–3154.

45. Capuani, S., Porcari, P., Fasano, F., Campanella, R. and Maraviglia, B. (2008). [10]B-editing [1]H-detection and ^{19}F MRI strategies to optimize boron neutron capture therapy. *Magn. Reson. Imaging* **26**, 987–993.

46. Porcari, P., Capuani, S., D'Amore, E., Lecce, M., Bella, A. L., Fasano, F., *et al.* (2009). In vivo ^{19}F MR imaging and spectroscopy for the BNCT optimization. *Appl. Radiat. Isot.* **67**, S365–S368.

47. Xiao, Y., Paudel, R., Liu, J., Ma, C., Zhang, Z. and Zhou, S. (2016). MRI contrast agents: Classification and application (Review). *Int. J. Mol. Med.* **38**, 1319–1326.

48. Nakamura, H., Fukuda, H., Girald, F., Kobayashi, T., Hiratsuka, J., Akaizawa, T., *et al.* (2000). In vivo evaluation of carborane gadolinium-DTPA complex as an MR imaging boron carrier. *Chem. Pharm. Bull.* **48**, 1034–1038.
49. Takahashi, K., Nakamura, H., Furumoto, S., Yamamoto, K., Fukuda, H., Matsumura, A., *et al.* (2005). Synthesis and in vivo biodistribution of BPA-Gd-DTPA complex as a potential MRI contrast carrier for neutron capture therapy. *Bioorg. Med. Chem.* **13**, 735–743.
50. Alberti, D., Deagostino, A., Toppino, A., Protti, N., Bortolussi, S., Altieri, S., *et al.* (2018). An innovative therapeutic approach for malignant mesothelioma treatment based on the use of Gd/boron multimodal probes for MRI guided BNCT. *J. Control. Release* **280**, 31–38.
51. Geninatti-Crich, S., Alberti, D., Szabo, I., Deagostino, A., Toppino, A., Barge, A., *et al.* (2011). MRI-guided neutron capture therapy by use of a dual gadolinium/boron agent targeted at tumour cells through upregulated low-density lipoprotein transporters. *Chem. Eur. J.* **17**, 8479–8486.
52. Ho, S. L., Yue, H., Tegafaw, T., Ahmad, M. Y., Liu, S., Nam, S. W., *et al.* (2022). Gadolinium neutron capture therapy (GdNCT) agents from molecular to nano: current status and perspectives. *ACS Omega* **7**, 2533–2553.
53. Mitchell, M. J., Billingsley, M. M., Haley, R. M., Wechsler, M. E., Peppas, N. A. and Langer, R. (2021). Engineering precision nanoparticles for drug delivery. *Nat. Rev. Drug. Discov.* **20**, 101–124.
54. Gao, S., Liu, X., Xu, T., Ma, X., Shen, Z., Wu, A., *et al.* (2013). Synthesis and characterization of Fe10BO3/Fe3O4/SiO2 and GdFeO3/Fe3O4/SiO2: Nanocomposites of biofunctional materials. *ChemistryOpen* **2**, 88–92.
55. Icten, O., Kose, D. A., Matissek, S. J., Misurelli, J. A., Elsawa, S. F., Hosmane, N. S., *et al.* (2018). Gadolinium borate and iron oxide bioconjugates: Nanocomposites of next generation with multifunctional applications. *Mater. Sci. Eng. C* **92**, 317–328.
56. Alberti, D., Protti, N., Toppino, A., Deagostino, A., Lanzardo, S., Bortolussi, S., *et al.* (2015). A theranostic approach based on the use of a dual boron/Gd agent to improve the efficacy of boron neutron capture therapy in the lung cancer treatment. *Nanomedicine* **11**, 741–750.
57. Alberti, D., Deagostino, A., Toppino, A., Protti, N., Bortolussi, S., Altieri, S., *et al.* (2018). An innovative therapeutic approach for malignant mesothelioma treatment based on the use of Gd/boron multimodal probes for MRI guided BNCT. *J. Control. Release* **280**, 31–38.
58. Kuthala, N., Vankayala, R., Li, Y. N., Chiang, C. S. and Hwang, K. C. (2017). Engineering novel targeted boron-10-enriched theranostic nanomedicine to combat against murine brain tumors via MR imaging-guided boron neutron capture therapy. *Adv. Mater.* **29**, 1700850.
59. Ishiwata, K., Ido, T., Mejia, A. A., Ichihashi, M. and Mishima, Y. (1991). Synthesis and radiation dosimetry of 4-borono-2-[¹⁸F]fluoro-D,L-phenylalanine: a target

compound for PET and boron neutron capture therapy. *Appl. Radiat. Isot.* **42**, 325–328.

60. Ishiwata, K., Shiono, M., Kubota, K., Yoshino, K., Hatazawa, J., Ido, T., *et al.* (1992). A unique in vivo assessment of 4-[^{10}B]borono-L-phenylalanine in tumor tissues for boron neutron capture therapy of malignant melanomas using positron emission tomography and 4-borono-2-[^{18}F]fluoro-L-phenylalanine. *Melanoma Res.* **2**, 171–180.

61. Kobayashi, T., Sakurai, Y. and Ishikawa, M. (2000). A noninvasive dose estimation system for clinical BNCT based on PG-SPECT-conceptual study and fundamental experiments using HPGe and CdTe semiconductor detectors. *Med. Phys.* **27**, 2124–2132.

62. Sakata, M., Oda, K., Toyohara, J., Ishii, K., Nariai, T. and Ishiwata, K. (2013). Direct comparison of radiation dosimetry of six PET tracers using human whole-body imaging and murine biodistribution studies. *Ann. Nucl. Med.* **27**, 285–296.

63. Kono, Y., Kurihara, H., Kawamoto, H., Yasui, N., Honda, N., Igaki, H., *et al.* (2017). Radiation absorbed dose estimates for ^{18}F-BPA PET. *Acta. Radiol.* **58**, 1094–1101.

64. Chadha, M., Capala, J., Coderre, J. A., Elowitz, E. H., Iwai, J., Joel, D. D., *et al.* (1998). Boron neutron-capture therapy (BNCT) for glioblastoma multiforme (GBM) using the epithermal neutron beam at the Brookhaven National Laboratory. *Int. J. Radiat. Oncol. Biol. Phys.* **40**, 829–834.

65. Suzuki, M., Kato, I., Aihara, T., Hiratsuka, J., Yoshimura, K., Niimi, M., *et al.* (2014). Boron neutron capture therapy outcomes for advanced or recurrent head and neck cancer. *J. Radiat. Res.* **55**, 146–153.

66. Miyashita, M., Miyatake, S.-I., Imahori, Y., Yokoyama, K., Kawabata, S., Kajimoto, Y., *et al.* (2008). Evaluation of fluoride-labeled boronophenylalanine-PET imaging for the study of radiation effects in patients with glioblastomas. *J. Neuro-oncol.* **89**, 239–246.

67. Miyatake, S., Kawabata, S., Hiramatsu, R., Kuroiwa, T., Suzuki, M., Kondo, N., *et al.* (2016). Boron neutron capture therapy for malignant brain tumors. *Neurol. Med. Chir.* **56**, 361–371.

68. Miyatake, S., Tamura, Y., Kawabata, S., Iida, K., Kuroiwa, T. and Ono, K. (2007). Boron neutron capture therapy for malignant tumors related to meningiomas. *Neurosurgery* **61**, 82–90.

69. Aihara, T., Hiratsuka, J., Morita, N., Uno, M., Sakurai, Y., Maruhashi, A., *et al.* (2006). First clinical case of boron neutron capture therapy for head and neck malignancies using ^{18}FBPA PET. *Head Neck* **28**, 850–855.

70. Aihara, T., Morita, N., Kamitani, N., Kumada, H., Ono, K., Hiratsuka, J., *et al.* (2014). Boron neutron capture therapy for advanced salivary gland carcinoma in head and neck. *Int. J. Clinic. Oncol.* **19**, 437–444.

71. Morita, T., Kur Ihara, H., Hiroi, K., Honda, N., Igaki, H., Hatazawa, J., *et al.* (2018). Dynamic changes in (18)F-borono-Lphenylalanine uptake in unresectable,

advanced, or recurrent squamous cell carcinoma of the head and neck and malignant melanoma during boron neutron capture therapy patient selection. *Radiat. Oncol.* **13**, 4.

72. Kankaanranta, L., Seppälä, T., Koivunoro, H., Saarilahti, K., Atula, T. and Collan, J. (2012). Boron neutron capture therapy in the treatment of locally recurred head-and-neck cancer: final analysis of a phase I/II trial. *Int. J. Radiat. Oncol. Biol. Phys.* **82**, e67–e75.
73. Wang, L. W., Wang, S. J., Chu, P. Y., Ho, C. Y., Jiang, S. H., Liu, Y. W. H., *et al.* (2011). BNCT for locally recurrent head and neck cancer: preliminary clinical experience from a phase I/II trial at Tsing Hua open-pool reactor. *Appl. Radiat. Isot.* **69**, 1803–1806.
74. Wang, L. W., Liu, Y. H. W., Chou, F. I. and Jiang, D-H. (2018). Clinical trials for treating recurrent head and neck cancer with boron neutron capture therapy using the Tsing–Hua open pool reactor. *Cancer Commun.* **38**, 37.
75. Lan, T. L., Chou, F. I., Lin, K. H., Pan, P. S., Lee, J. C., Huang, W. S., *et al.* (2020). Using salvage boron neutron capture therapy (BNCT) for recurrent malignant brain tumors in Taiwan. *Appl. Radiat. Isot.* **160**, 109105.
76. Chen, Y. W., Lee, Y. Y., Lin, C. F., Pan, P. S., Chen, J. K., Wang, C. W., *et al.* (2021). Salvage boron neutron capture therapy for malignant brain tumor patients in compliance with emergency and compassionate use: Evaluation of 34 cases in Taiwan. *Biology* **10**, 334.
77. Chen, Y. W., Lee, Y. Y., Lin, C. F., Huang, T. Y., Ke, S. H., Mu, P. F., *et al.* (2022). Compassionate treatment of brainstem tumors with boron neutron capture therapy: a case series. *Life* **12**, 566.
78. Kato, I., Fujita, Y., Maruhashi, A., Kumada, H., Ohmae, M., Kirihata, M., *et al.* (2009). Effectiveness of boron neutron capture therapy for recurrent head and neck malignancies. *Appl. Radiat. Isot.* **67**, S37–S42.
79. Wu, C. Y., Lin, J. J., Chang, W. Y., Hsieh, C. Y., Wu, C. C., Chen, H. S., *et al.* (2019). Development of theranostic active-targeting boron-containing gold nanoparticles for boron neutron capture therapy (BNCT). *Colloids Surf. B Biointerfaces* **183**, 110387.
80. Pulagam, K. R., Gona, K. B., Gómez-Vallejo, V., Meijer, J., Zilberfain, C., Estrela-Lopis, I., *et al.* (2019). Gold nanoparticles as boron carriers for boron neutron capture therapy: synthesis, radiolabelling and in vivo evaluation. *Molecules* **24**, 3609.
81. Feiner, I. V. J., Pulagam, K. R., Gómez-Vallejo, V., Zamacola, K., Baz, Z., Caffarel, M. M., *et al.* (2020). Therapeutic pretargeting with gold nanoparticles as drug candidates for boron neutron capture therapy. *Part. Part. Syst. Charact.* **37**, 2000200.
82. Iguchi, Y., Michiue, H., Kitamatsu, M., Hayashi, Y., Takenaka, F., Nishiki, T., *et al.* (2015). Tumor-specific delivery of BSH-3R for boron neutron capture therapy and positron emission tomography imaging in a mouse brain tumor model. *Biomaterials* **56**, 10–17.

83. Kumar, N., Singh DNB, R. K. R., Dutta, D. and Kheruka, S. C. (2017). Lu-177 – A noble tracer: future of personalized radionuclide therapy. *Clin. Oncol.* **2**, 1249.
84. Kalot, G., Godard, A., Busser, B., Pliquett, J., Broekgaarden, M., Motto-Ros, V., *et al.* (2020). Aza-BODIPY: A new vector for enhanced theranostic boron neutron capture therapy applications. *Cells* **9**, 1953.
85. Zhao, F., Hu, K., Shao, C. and Jin, G. (2021). Original boron cluster covalent with poly-zwitterionic BODIPYs for boron neutron capture therapy agent. *Polym. Test.* **100**, 107269.
86. Guseva, G., Antina, E., Berezin, M., Lisovskaya, S., Pavelyev, R., Kayumov, A., *et al.* (2020). Spectroscopic and in vitro investigations of boron(III) complex with meso-4-methoxycarbonylpropylsubstituted dipyrromethene for fluorescence bio-imaging applications. *Molecules* **25**, 4541.
87. Hudson, R. and Boyle, R. W. (2004). Strategies for selective delivery of photody-namic sensitisers to biological targets. *J. Porphyr. Phthalocyanines* **8**, 954–975.
88. Chen, X. and Drain, M. C. (2004). Photodynamic therapy using carbohydrate conjugated porphyrins. *Drug Design Rev.* **1**, 215–234.
89. Wei, W. H., Wang, Z., Mizuno, T., Cortez, C., Fu, L., Sirisawad, M., *et al.* (2006). New polyethyleneglycol-functionalized texaphyrins: synthesis and in vitro biologi-cal studies. *Dalton. Trans.* **(16)**, 1934–1942.
90. Smilowitz, H. M., Slatkin, D. N., Micca, P. L. and Miura, M. (2013). Microlocalization of lipophilic porphyrins: Non-toxic enhancers of boron neu-tron-capture therapy, *Int. J. Radiat. Biol.* **89**, 611–617,
91. Shi, Y., Li, J., Zhang, Z., Duan, D., Zhang, Z., Liu, H., *et al.* (2018). Tracing boron with fluorescence and positron emission tomography imaging of boronated porphyrin nanocomplex for imaging-guided boron neutron capture therapy. *ACS Appl. Mater. Interfaces.* **10**, 43387–43395.
92. Bregadze, V. I., Sivaev, I. B., Gabel, D. and Wöhrle, D. (2001). Polyhedral boron derivatives of porphyrins and phthalocyanines. *J. Porphyr. Phthalocyanines* **5**, 767–781.
93. Dubey, R., Kushal, S., Mollard, A., Vojtovich, L., Oh, P., Levin, M. D., *et al.* (2015). Tumor targeting, trifunctional dendritic wedge. *Bioconjug. Chem.* **26**, 78–89.

https://doi.org/10.1142/9789811268038_0005

Chapter 5

Developments in Neutron Sources for Boron Neutron Capture Therapy

Xiyin Zhang,* Yusheng Lin

Shenzhen HEC Industrial Development Co. Ltd.

Abstract

This chapter describes the development of boron neutron capture therapy (BNCT) from several technical aspects, including the neutron source, dosimetry and the treatment process. The principle of BNCT to kill tumor cells is mainly based on the nuclear reaction between thermal neutrons and boron. The energy generated by this nuclear reaction will destroy the double helix structure of DNA in the nucleus, making it impossible to repair and causing apoptosis of the whole cell. While the boron drug is the protagonist, the development and application of neutron sources and nuclear-related technologies are also a crucial aspect. The differences between the two types of neutron source, reactor-based and accelerator-based, as well as the key components and related technologies of these neutron sources are discussed. Three typical BNCT facilities in the world are also introduced. An entire section is dedicated to dosimetry, as accurate dose assessment and calculation are the key to the success of BNCT. The chapter is completed by a step-by-step explanation of the treatment planning system and treatment process.

Keywords: neutron, cross-section, neutron source, accelerator, dosimetry, treatment planning system.

Boron neutron capture therapy (BNCT) is a technique that was designed to selectively target high linear energy transfer (LET)[1] heavy

---

[1] LET is the average (radiation) energy deposited per unit path length along the track of an ionizing particle. Its units are keV/μm.
*Corresponding author.

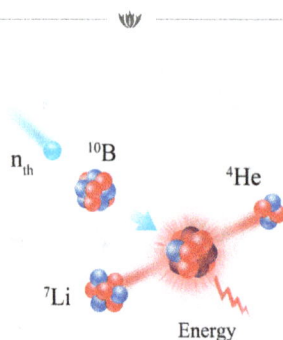

Figure 5.1 The nuclear reaction that describes the foundation of BNCT.

charged particle radiation to tumors at the cellular level. BNCT is different from the conventional radiation therapy that involves the use of high-energy X ray or electron beams, which is described as having a low LET since the energy deposition in tissues as ionizations are spatially infrequent. In addition, BNCT is a binary form of radiation therapy with low-energy neutrons captured by boron compounds concentrated in the tumor tissue, where ^{10}B briefly becomes ^{11}B, then immediately disintegrates into an energetic α particle with a recoiling ^{7}Li. The nuclear reaction is described in Eq. (5.1) and Figure 5.1.

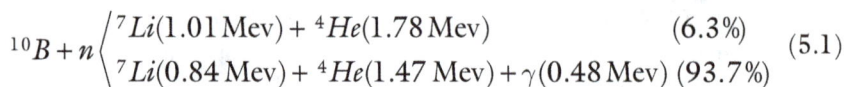

$$^{10}B + n \begin{cases} ^{7}Li(1.01\,\text{Mev}) + {}^{4}He(1.78\,\text{Mev}) & (6.3\%) \\ ^{7}Li(0.84\,\text{Mev}) + {}^{4}He(1.47\,\text{Mev}) + \gamma(0.48\,\text{Mev}) & (93.7\%) \end{cases} \quad (5.1)$$

The $^{10}B(n, \alpha)^{7}Li$ nuclear reaction can release ^{7}Li and α particles in the first excited state with a total energy of 2.79 MeV or ^{7}Li and α particles in the ground state with a total energy of 2.31 MeV. Regressing from the first excited state to the ground state will release a γ photon of 0.48 MeV. Since both the α particle and the ^{7}Li are charged heavy nuclei, they have a short range (5 μm for ^{7}Li and 8 μm for the α particle) and a high LET (200–300 keV/μm), which translates to a high relative biological effectiveness (RBE)[2], as all their energy will be deposited in a cell (10 μm).

---

[2] RBE is a unitless quantity that is calculated for a specific radiation (A) of interest. It is the ratio of the dose of a reference radiation required to produce a specific level of response to the dose of radiation (A) producing an equal response. All variables, except radiation quality, are held as constant as possible. There is a consensus that the RBE of X-rays (from 0.1 to 3 MeV) is equal to 1, whatever the energy or dose rate of the beam.

There are two necessary conditions for this therapy to be effective: 1) the boron compound must be non-toxic, low in normal tissues, and tumor-concentrated, with a sufficient number of ^{10}B deposited into each tumor cell; 2) low-energy neutrons, which are thermal neutrons, must be sufficiently targeted into each tumor cell.

Two different neutron beams are commonly used in BNCT: thermal beams where therapeutic benefit is limited to shallow depths, and epithermal beams; with multiple beams, the effect may extend to 8–10 cm.

Both types of beams include contributions by fast, epithermal, and thermal neutrons, as well as γ rays. Before discussing the practicalities of current and potential neutron sources, how to modify reactors and how to adjust beams, it is first necessary to establish the beam characteristics desired for BNCT.

For BNCT, an adequate thermal neutron field has to be generated in the boron-labeled tumor cells within a prescribed target volume. This means that for target volumes well below the surface, epithermal beam is usually the best, while for target volumes near the surface, thermal beam is sufficient.

Figure 5.2 shows that an epithermal neutron beam entering tissue produces a radiation field with a maximum thermal flux at a depth of 2–3 cm, which drops exponentially thereafter. Beam penetration can be increased, especially for small beam sizes, by increasing the average energy of the epithermal neutrons and by increasing the forward direction of the beam. The thermal flux of the thermal neutron beam falls off exponentially from the surface compared to the epithermal beam that shows a skin-sparing effect.

Therefore, thermal neutron irradiation has been used in the treatment for melanoma in the skin, as well as for glioma in open craniotomy. In general, however, the current trend in treating patients with brain tumors is to use epithermal neutron beams.

On the other hand, radiobiology research for BNCT requires both thermal and epithermal beams. Clinical facilities are available to study the effects of epithermal irradiation, but pure thermal neutron fields are preferred when studying the effect of boron carrier compounds using cell cultures or small animals. Before describing the neutron sources for BNCT, the basics of the neutron are introduced.

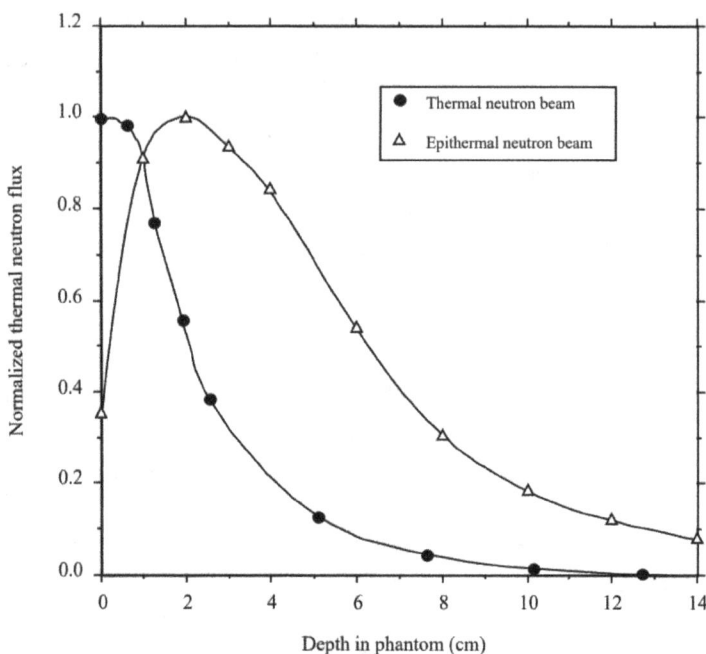

Figure 5.2 Comparison of flux-depth distributions for thermal and epithermal neutrons [1].

5.1 The Neutron

Matter in the universe is composed of molecules and atoms, and atoms are composed of a nucleus and extranuclear electrons. Protons and neutrons make up the nucleus of an atom. Neutrons are neutral particles, *i.e.*, have no net electric charge, which is why they are named as "neutron". The neutron was discovered by James Chadwick of the Cavendish Laboratory at Cambridge University in 1932.

The mass of the neutron is $1.6749286 \times 10^{-27}$ kg, slightly heavier than that of a proton which is $1.672621637 \times 10^{-27}$ kg. The neutron used to be listed as a member of the elementary particles (a term in physics that refers to the smallest or most basic unit for composing matter). However, in the current Standard Model theory, the neutron is found to be a composite particle composed of two down quarks and one up quark (a quark is one of the elementary or fundamental particles).

5.1.1 *Discovery of the Neutron*

The discovery of the existence and properties of neutrons was a pivotal moment for extraordinary developments in atomic physics in the first half of the 20th century. Ernest Rutherford, a physicist of the Cavendish Laboratory at Cambridge University, proposed a description of the structure of atoms in 1911, now known as the Rutherford model, Rutherford atomic model, nuclear atomic model or planetary model of the atom. The atomic structure model posited that all positive charges and nearly all the mass of an atom are concentrated in a tiny and dense core region, called a nucleus, and electrons travel in circular orbits around the nucleus, just like a planet revolves around the sun. The nucleus is positively charged and the electrons are negatively charged. But the Achilles heel of Rutherford's atomic model is that the electric field force between positive and negative charges cannot satisfy the requirement of stability. It cannot explain how the electrons stay outside the nucleus stably. According to the classical electromagnetic theory, the electrostatic attraction between the positively charged nucleus and the negatively charged electron causes the electron to generate a centripetal acceleration, which makes the electron rotate around the nucleus. The electron will emit electromagnetic radiation when it gains acceleration, and this electromagnetic radiation will consume energy. As a result of the continuous consumption of energy, the trajectory of the electron will become smaller and smaller, and finally it will inevitably fall on the nucleus which will disintegrate. But in reality, atoms are very stable.

At the time, it was known through experiments that for most atoms, the atomic number Z of the nucleus is numerically half or less than the atomic mass number A. This phenomenon does not satisfy the law of conservation of mass number. Therefore, Rutherford first predicted the existence of neutrons in the Bakerian Lecture of the Royal Society in 1920. He suggested that a neutrally charged particle which is about the same mass as a proton might exist in the nucleus. Rutherford's student James Chadwick began his experimental exploration of neutrons in 1921.

An experimental observation in 1930 brought a breakthrough (Figure 5.3). It was found that unusually penetrating radiation was generated if the very energetic α particles emitted from polonium

119

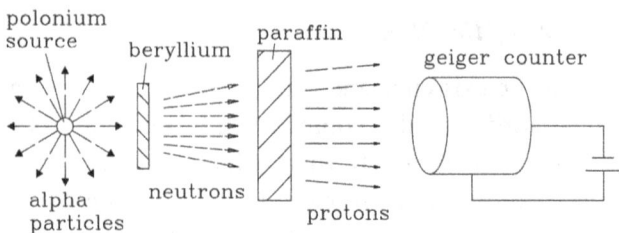

Figure 5.3   The α particles emitted from polonium bombard certain light elements, and generated unusually penetrating radiation.

bombard certain light elements, specifically beryllium, boron, or lithium. Since the electric field could not influence this radiation, it was presumed as γ rays with more penetrating power. When a paraffin target with this radiation was bombarded, it emitted protons with an energy of about 5.3 MeV as shown in Figure 5.3. These experimental phenomena were difficult to interpret at that time. Chadwick studied and doubted that it was γ rays. He bombarded nitrogen nuclei with the same radiation again. If it was γ rays, the calculated energies of the two experimental phenomena by Compton scattering would contradict each other. So obviously it was not γ rays, but a new kind of neutral particle.

What to do next was to determine the mass of this neutral particle. Chadwick bombarded boron with α particles and analyzed the interaction of the neutral particles with nitrogen. The boron and nitrogen targets were partly chosen because their masses were well known. He used instruments to measure the velocities of the hydrogen and nitrogen nuclei that were bombarded out, from which he deduced the mass of the new particle through the law of conservation of momentum. Chadwick also experimented with other substances, and the result was that the mass of this neutral particle was about the same as that of a hydrogen nucleus. Since this particle had no charge, it was called a neutron. Later, more precise experiments determined that the mass of the neutron is very similar to that of the proton, only about one thousandth greater. Chadwick wrote his research as a paper "The Presence of Neutrons", which was published in the *Proceedings of the Royal Society*. In 1935, he won the Nobel Prize in Physics for this discovery.

5.1.2 Properties of the Neutron

The nucleus accounts for 99.9% of the atomic mass. Although the chemical properties of an atom are determined by the number of protons, without neutrons it is impossible to form elements other than hydrogen, which has only one proton, due to the repulsion between positively charged protons. The competition between two fundamental interactions determines the stability of the nucleus. Protons and neutrons are attracted to each other by the strong nuclear force (one of the four fundamental forces in nature; the other three are gravity, electromagnetism and the weak nuclear force). On the other hand, protons repel each other by electric force due to their positive charges. The attraction between neutrons and protons helps counteract the electrical repulsion between the protons.

Due to the power of the short-range nuclear force, the nuclear binding energy of a nucleon (the energy required to break an atomic nucleus into its component parts) is more than seven orders of magnitude larger than the electromagnetic energy of bound electrons in atoms. Consequently, nuclear reactions (such as nuclear fission or fusion) have a greater energy density than that of chemical reactions.

Key properties of neutrons are summarized as follows:

- Mean square radius of a neutron is ~0.8×10^{-15} m.
- The mass of the neutron is 939.565 MeV/c^2 or about $1.6749286 \times 10^{-27}$ kg.
- Neutron charge: zero (q < 1×10^{-27} e).
- Free neutrons are unstable and undergo β decay (β decay is a type of radioactive decay involving the emission of β particles, which are electrons or positrons).
- The mean lifetime of a free neutron is 882 seconds (*i.e.*, the half-life is 611 seconds).
- Neutrons cannot directly cause ionization. Neutrons can only indirectly ionize matter.
- Neutrons can travel extremely long distances in the air without any interaction. Neutron radiation has strong penetrability.
- The wavelength of thermal or cold neutrons is similar to the atomic spacing. They can be used in neutron diffraction experiments to determine the atomic and/or magnetic structure of a material.

5.1.3 *Free Neutrons*

Free neutrons are neutrons that exist outside of an atomic nucleus. While neutrons can be stable when bound within the nucleus, free neutrons are unstable and they decay. Scientists have used the "bottle" method to make the most precise measurement of a neutron's lifetime. The new results report a neutron lifetime of 877.75 seconds (about 14.629 minutes) with an uncertainty of 0.039% (about 0.005 minutes). This result is consistent with theoretical calculations and is twice as accurate as previous measurements. The half-life of a free neutron is affected by the weak nuclear force, and after decay a neutron becomes a proton, an electron and an electron antineutrino (the antimatter counterpart of the neutrino, a particle with no charge and little or no mass), and the proton and electron form a hydrogen atom. The half-life of a free neutron is about 611 seconds (10.3 minutes). Because they decay in this way, neutrons do not exist in nature in their free state, except among other high-energy particles in cosmic rays.

Free neutrons can be classified according to their kinetic energy. This energy is usually expressed in electron volts (eV). The term temperature can also describe the energy that represents the thermal equilibrium between neutrons and a medium with a certain temperature.

Common classifications based on kinetic energies are as follows:

- *Cold Neutrons:* 0 eV ~ 0.025 eV. A cold neutron stays in thermal equilibrium with very cold surroundings such as liquid deuterium. This spectrum is used for neutron scattering experiments.
- *Thermal Neutrons:* A thermal neutron stays in thermal equilibrium with the surrounding particles at Normal Temperature and Pressure (NTP). It means that the average kinetic energy of thermal neutrons is the same as that of any gas atom at 20°C. Their energy distribution is given by the Maxwell-Boltzmann formula. The most probable energy at room temperature (20°C) is 0.025 eV. The average energy is 0.038 eV. The velocity is approximately 2.2 km/s.
- *Epithermal Neutrons:* 0.025 eV ~ 1 eV.
- *Slow Neutrons:* 1 eV ~ 10 eV.

- *Resonance Neutrons:* 10 eV ~ 300 eV. At resonance energy, the cross-section can reach a peak value more than 100 times higher than the base value of the cross-section and the neutron capture significantly exceeds the possibility of fission.
- *Intermediate Neutrons:* 300 eV ~ 1 MeV.
- *Fast Neutrons:* 1 MeV ~ 20 MeV. Neutrons of kinetic energy greater than 1 MeV (~15,000 km/s) are usually generated by nuclear processes such as nuclear fission or (α, n) reactions.[3]
- *Relativistic Neutrons:* >20 MeV.

In many cases, this fine division of neutron energies is unnecessary. They can be roughly divided into three energy ranges:

- *Thermal neutrons:* 0.025 eV ~ 0.5 eV.
- *Epithermal neutrons:* 0.5 eV ~ 10 keV.
- *Fast neutrons:* 10 keV ~ 10 MeV.

---

[3] In a nuclear reaction, the particle used to bombard the nucleus is called the incident particle or the bombarding particle, the bombarded nucleus is called the target nucleus, the particle emitted by the nuclear reaction is called the outgoing particle, and the nucleus generated by the reaction is called the residual nucleus or product nucleus. The nuclear reaction in which the incoming particle "a" bombards the target nucleus "A", emits the outgoing particle "b" and generates the remaining nucleus "B" can be expressed by the following equation:

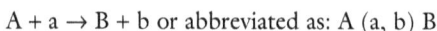

$$A + a \rightarrow B + b \text{ or abbreviated as: } A\,(a, b)\,B$$

According to the different incident particles, nuclear reactions can be divided into three categories:

(1) Neutron nuclear reactions, such as elastic scattering of neutrons (n, n), inelastic scattering (n, v2), radiation capture of neutrons (n, γ), nuclear reactions that emit charged particles (n, p), (n, α), *etc.*, neutron fission reactions (n, f), and nuclear reactions that emit two or more particles (n, 2n), (n, pn), *etc.*;

(2) Charged particle nuclear reactions, such as nuclear reactions caused by protons (p, γ), (p, n), (p, p), (p, π2), (p, α), (p, 2n), *etc.*, deuterons (d, n), (d, p), (d, α), *etc.*, α-particles (α, n), (α, 2n), (α, p), *etc.*, and nuclear reactions caused by heavy ions (^{12}C, ^{4}n), (^{22}Ne, ^{6}n), *etc.*;

(3) Photonuclear reaction, that is, the nuclear reaction caused by photons, such as (γ, n), (γ, p), (γ, α), (γ, f) and so on.

5.1.4 *Interactions of Neutrons with Matter*

Neutrons are uncharged and can travel appreciable distances in straight lines through matter without interaction. Only when they collide with the nucleus to disperse in a new direction or be absorbed will they deviate from the original path. The electrons around the nucleus and the electric field generated by the positively charged nucleus will not affect the flight of neutrons. In short, neutrons collide with nuclei, not atoms.

Neutrons can interact with an atomic nucleus through:

(1) Elastic Scattering Reaction

Elastic scattering occurs when a neutron collides with an atomic nucleus without being absorbed by or exciting the nucleus. In elastic scattering, the total kinetic energy of the neutron-nucleus system does not change. The total kinetic energy is conserved and the energy loss by the neutron is equal to the kinetic energy of the recoil nucleus.

Elastic scattering is usually the primary physical interaction of neutrons traveling through matter, and the primary mechanism for fast neutron dose delivery to tissue. If the mass of the nucleus is low, such as hydrogen or carbon, neutrons can transfer most of their energy to the nucleus. In this case, the mass of the nucleus can be inferred by measuring the energy and direction of the scattered neutrons. The phenomenon of elastic scattering is often used to moderate fast neutrons for shielding, and can also be used to detect fast neutrons.

(2) Inelastic Scattering Reaction

In inelastic neutron scattering, the energy and momentum exchange between the incident neutron and the sample causes the direction and magnitude of the neutron's wave vector to change. This type of scattering is a commonly used technique in condensed matter research, which is used to study atomic and molecular motion, magnetic field and crystal field excitation.

(3) Neutron Absorption

The absorption reactions are nuclear reactions where the neutron is completely absorbed, and the compound nucleus is formed. The most important absorption reactions are divided by the exit channel into two following reactions:

a)   Radiative Capture

Radiative capture is a reaction where the incident neutron is completely absorbed, and the compound nucleus is formed. Then the compound nucleus decays to the ground state by γ emission. This is referred to as a capture reaction, also as a radiative capture or (n, γ) reaction.[4] This process can occur at all incident neutron energies, but the probability of the interaction largely depends on the incident neutron energy and the target energy.

b)   Nuclear Fission

Nuclear fission is the splitting of atomic nuclei into multiple parts (lighter nuclei), which usually emit γ rays, free neutrons and other subatomic particles as by-products. The fission of heavy elements is an exothermic reaction, which can release a large amount of energy. Nuclear fission can be used and controlled by a chain reaction: the free neutrons released by each fission event can trigger more events, thus releasing more neutrons and causing more fission.

The probability of particular interaction between an incident neutron and a target nucleus is described in terms of quantities known as cross-sections. It must be noted the probability does not depend on real target dimensions. It enables the calculation of the reaction rate in conjunction with the neutron flux. The standard unit for measuring the cross-section (σ) is the barn, equal to 10^{-24} cm^2 or 10^{-28} m^2.

The cross-section is variable and depends on:

- Target nucleus (hydrogen, boron, uranium, *etc.*). Each isotope has its own set of cross-sections.
- The type of nuclear reaction (capture, fission, *etc.*).
- Neutron energy (cold neutrons, thermal neutrons, *etc.*). For a given target nucleus and reaction type, the cross-section largely depends on the neutron energy. In common cases, the cross-section at low energies is usually much larger than at high energies.
- The relative angle between the incident neutron and the target nucleus.
- Target energy (temperature of target material). This dependency is not so obvious.

---

[4] BNCT is the abbreviation of Boron Neutron Capture Therapy, which clearly shows that it is a kind of capture reaction, or (n, γ) reaction.

In the human body, four elements, namely, oxygen, carbon, hydrogen, and nitrogen, are considered the most essential elements. Oxygen is the most abundant element in the human body, accounting for approximately 61% of a person's mass. In BNCT, the nuclear reaction between thermal neutrons and ^{10}B is dominant. The absorption cross-section is 3,848 barns, which is quite a large number compared to the cross-section of other common elements constituting the tissues, such as ^1H (30 barns), ^{14}N (10.55 barns), ^{13}C (6 barns), and ^{16}O (3.9 barns) [2].

5.1.5 *Neutron Sources*

Neutrons are very abundant in the universe, accounting for almost half of all visible matter. But on earth, neutrons only appear as bound particles in atoms. Therefore, free neutrons for research, industrial or medical applications need to be generated by nuclear reactions. A neutron source is any device that emits neutrons.

There are several kinds of neutron sources described below.

(1) Large-Sized Devices

• Neutron Reactors
In 1939, Hahn and Strassman discovered nuclear fission caused by the capture of a slow neutron in uranium-235 (Figure 5.4). The fact that several neutrons are emitted when fission occurs indicates that a self-sustaining chain reaction may be possible. When the output of a nuclear reaction causes more nuclear reactions, a nuclear chain reaction will occur. These chain reactions are almost always a series of fission events, releasing excess neutrons. These excess neutrons can continue to cause more fission events, hence the name chain reaction. The world's first man-made nuclear reactor entered a critical state on December 2, 1942.

There are nuclei that can undergo fission on their own spontaneously, but only certain nuclei, like uranium-235, uranium-233, and plutonium-239, which will release neutrons when they split, can sustain a fission chain reaction. Uranium-235, which exists as 0.7% of naturally occurring uranium, undergoes nuclear fission with thermal neutrons, generating an

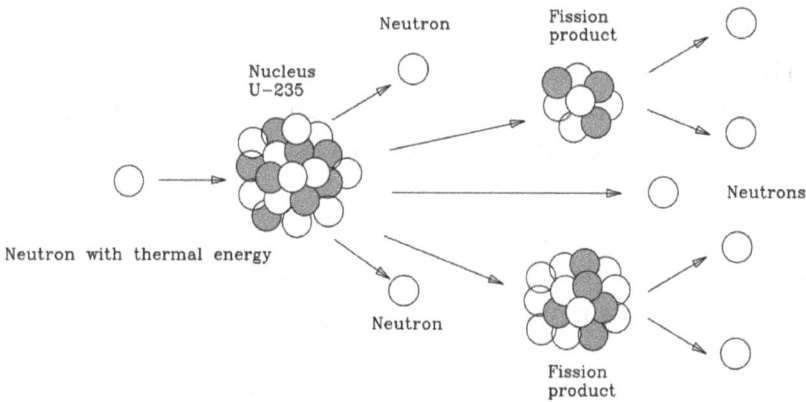

Figure 5.4   Schematic of fission processes.

average of 2.4 fast neutrons and the release of about 180 MeV of energy per fission. The free neutrons released from each fission play a very important role as triggers for reactions, but they can also be used for other purposes. For example, a neutron is needed to trigger further fission. Some free neutrons (assuming 0.5 neutrons/fission) are absorbed by other materials, but excessive neutrons (0.9 neutrons/fission) will leave the surface of the reactor core and can be used as a neutron source.

• Fusion Systems
Nuclear fusion, the combining of the heavy isotopes of hydrogen, where two or more atomic nuclei (*e.g.*, D+T) collide at very high energy and fuse together, also has the potential to generate large quantities of neutrons.

• Spallation Sources
A spallation source consists of a high-power accelerator that brings protons with energy greater than 0.5 GeV into a heavy metal target, such as mercury or tungsten. These metals will "spall off" free neutrons on impact. They are the brightest neutron sources used for research in the world. As accelerators can easily generate pulses, spallation sources are usually pulsed neutron sources, which is different from most reactors that produce neutrons constantly.

(2) Medium-Sized Devices

- High-Energy Bremsstrahlung Photoneutron / Photofission Systems
Neutrons are generated when photons above the nuclear binding energy of a substance are incident on that substance, causing it to emit a neutron or undergo fission.

- Light Ion Accelerators
Conventional particle accelerators with hydrogen (H), deuterium (D), or tritium (T) ion sources can be used to generate neutrons by (p, n)/ (d, n)/(t, n) reactions using target materials of deuterium, tritium, lithium, beryllium, and other low-Z materials. Typically, these accelerators operate at voltages under 1 MeV.[5]

(3) Small-Sized Devices

- Neutron Generators
The fusion of deuterium and tritium can generate neutrons. It is easy to achieve in the laboratory with a modest 100 kV accelerator for deuterium ions bombarding a tritium target. Continuous neutron sources of about 10^{11} n/s can be achieved relatively simply.

- Radioisotope Source: (α, n) Reaction
In certain light isotopes, there are neutrons in the nucleus with weak binding energy, which can be released when the compound nucleus formed following α particle bombardment decays. This reaction produces a weak neutron source with an energy spectrum similar to that of a fission source, and is now used in portable neutron sources.

- Radioisotope Source: (γ, n) Reaction
This kind of source generates monoenergetic neutrons, unlike (α, n) sources.

- Radioisotope Source: Spontaneous Fission
Certain isotopes undergo spontaneous fission with the emission of neutrons. The most commonly used spontaneous fission source is the radioisotope californium-252. Cf-252 and other spontaneous fission

---

[5] Most accelerator-based BNCT facilities use light ion accelerators.

neutron sources are produced by irradiating uranium or another transuranic element in a nuclear reactor.

5.1.6 *Neutron Moderators*

Neutron moderators are materials that can be used to slow down the fast neutrons, turning them into thermal neutrons to sustain the fission chain reaction. The moderation of the neutrons makes them more easily absorbed by fissile nuclei, creating more fission events (see Figure 5.5).

A very specific set of properties is required for moderation materials. First, the moderator should not absorb neutrons, which means that the moderator should have a low neutron absorption cross-section. The moderator should then be able to slow down the neutrons to an acceptable speed. Therefore, an ideal moderator's neutron scattering cross-section should be very high. The elastic collision occurs between neutrons and nucleus, which means that when the size of the nucleus

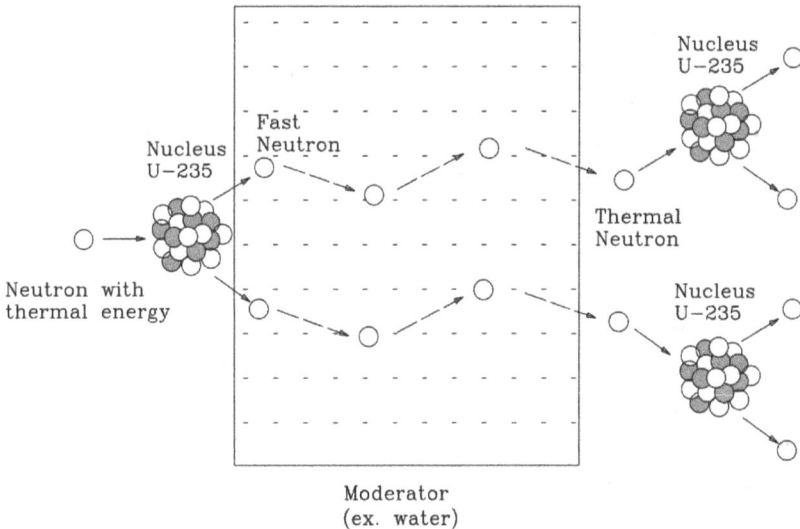

Figure 5.5 Thermal neutrons undergo nuclear fission with uranium-235 to generate fast neutrons. The moderator will then slow down these fast neutrons to thermal neutrons, which can sustain the nuclear chain reaction. When this process is repeated, the fission events double each time.

Table 5.1   Properties of common neutron moderators.

	Neutron Scattering Cross-Section (σ_s) in barns	Neutron Absorption Cross-Section (σ_a) in barns
Light water (H$_2$O)	49	0.66
Heavy water (D$_2$O)	10.6	0.0013
Graphite (C)	4.7	0.0035

in the moderator is closer to that of neutrons, the energy transfer is more obvious and the speed is slower. For this reason, smaller atomic number elements are more efficient moderators.

Several common moderator materials used in reactors are introduced below, including light water, heavy water and graphite. These materials have different moderating abilities and costs. Table 5.1 shows their neutron absorption cross-sections and scattering cross-sections.

Many reactors use light water as neutron moderator because it contains large amounts of hydrogen atoms. The hydrogen atom works well as a neutron moderator because its mass is almost the same as that of a neutron. It means that the elastic collision can significantly reduce the speed of neutrons due to the conservation laws of energy and momentum. Light water is no different from regular water. It is abundant in nature and quite cheap. One disadvantage is that hydrogen has a high neutron absorption cross-section because it can form deuterium. Therefore, light water is used together with enriched fuel. Enriched uranium fuel has a high uranium concentration and can sustain the chain reaction in the case that the number of neutrons is reduced due to absorption by light water. However, it is expensive to build a uranium isotope separation plant or enriched uranium plant. Reactors using light water are called light water reactors, including the pressurized water reactor, the boiling water reactor, and the supercritical water-cooled reactor.

The reason heavy water is used as neutron moderator in reactors is that its scattering cross-section for neutrons is large, like light water. But because it contains deuterium atoms, the neutron absorption cross-section is much lower than that of light water. The main disadvantage to the use of heavy water is its high cost of production. Reactors that use heavy water include the CANDU designs and the pressurized heavy water reactor.

Graphite, which requires very high purity to be effective, is also used as moderator. The cost of high-purity graphite is very low. In addition, it has thermal stability and good thermal conductivity. However, at high temperature, graphite will still react with oxygen and carbon dioxide in the reactor, which will reduce the effectiveness of its moderation. Another potential issue with using graphite as moderator is its ability to oxidize in the presence of air, and its low strength and density which could cause it to change dimensions in the reactor. Reactors that use graphite moderator include the RBMK and pebble bed reactors.

5.1.7 Shielding of Neutrons

In radiation protection, there are three ways to protect people from or lessen harm from identified radiation sources:

(1) *Limiting Exposure Time.* Radiation exposure is directly dependent on the time people spend near the radiation source. The dose can be reduced by limiting exposure time.

(2) *Keep Safe Distance.* Radiation exposure depends on the distance from the radiation source. The radiation dose drops sharply with increasing distance from the radiation source.

(3) *Shielding.* Radiation shielding usually consists of barriers of water, concrete, or lead. The shielding to be used depends on the specific radiation type to be shielded.

The following three characteristics of neutrons are critical for neutron shielding:

(1) Neutrons are not charged. Therefore, they are not affected or stopped by electric fields. This makes neutrons highly penetrating.

(2) It is difficult to slow down neutrons by scattering with heavy nuclei, let alone absorb fast neutrons. Therefore, lead is very ineffective in blocking neutron radiation because neutrons are not charged and can simply pass through dense materials.

(3) The absorption of neutrons triggers certain other nuclear reactions (*e.g.*, radiative capture or even fission), along with many other types of radiation. In short, neutrons activate other substances, making them radioactive. Therefore, we must also shield the other types of radiation.

The ideal materials for shielding neutrons must have the following characteristics:

(1) Slow down neutrons (the same principle as neutron moderation) It can be achieved through materials containing low atomic number, such as water, polyethylene and concrete.

(2) Absorb thermal neutrons
Thermal neutrons are easily captured and absorbed by materials with high neutron capture cross-sections, such as boron, lithium, or cadmium whose capture cross-section with thermal neutrons is several thousands of barns. Only a thin layer of such material is enough to shield thermal neutrons. The capture cross-section of hydrogen and thermal neutron is only 0.3 barns. This is far from enough, but it can be compensated by setting the sufficient thickness of the water shield.

(3) Shield the accompanying radiation
In the case of cadmium shield, the absorption of neutrons is accompanied by strong emission of γ rays. Therefore, additional shield is required to block the γ rays. But for boron, that's not a big deal. Boron nuclei absorb neutrons without intense γ emission, and thus boron-containing materials are often used for neutron shielding.

Water is an effective and common neutron shield, but not an acceptable γ ray shield. Water can perfectly moderate neutrons, but as neutrons are absorbed by hydrogen nuclei, high-energy secondary γ rays will be generated. These γ rays have strong penetrability to substances, and therefore they increase requirements on the thickness of the water shield. Since boric acid is soluble in water, boric acid can be added to water as a very effective neutron shielding solution

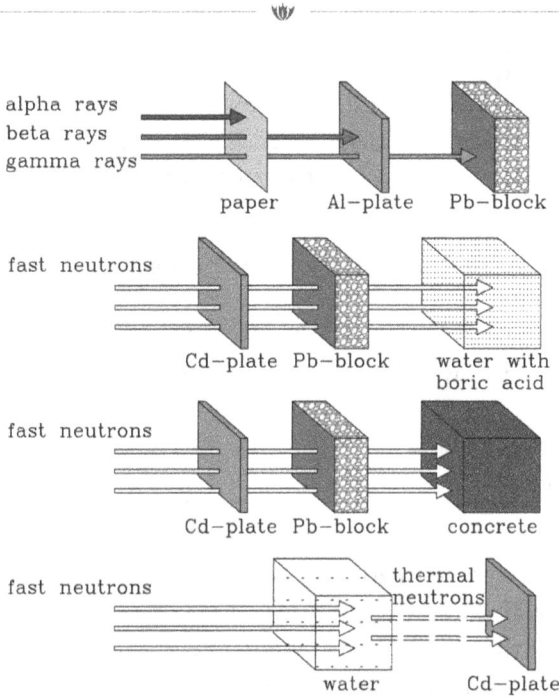

Figure 5.6 Water as a neutron shield.

(Figure 5.6), but results in another problem that is corrosion of construction materials.

The most commonly used neutron shield in nuclear engineering is concrete shielding. Concrete is also a high hydrogen material, but unlike water, concrete has a higher density for secondary γ shielding and requires little maintenance. Because concrete is a mixture of several different materials, its composition is not constant. Generally speaking, concrete is divided into "normal" concrete and "heavy" concrete. Heavy concrete has a higher density than normal concrete ($\sim$2,300 kg/m^3). Heavy concrete provides very effective protection.

5.2 Neutron Sources for BNCT

One of the principal conditions for BNCT to be successful is there must be a sufficient number of low-energy (thermal/epithermal) neutrons

Table 5.2 IAEA's recommendation on beam characteristics of the neutron sources for BNCT.

Parameter	Nomenclature	IAEA Recommendation
Epithermal beam intensity	Φ_{epi} (n/cm^{2}s)	$>1.0 \times 10^9$
Fast neutron dose per epithermal neutron	D_f/Φ_{epi} (Gy·cm^2/n)	$<2.0 \times 10^{-13}$
γ dose per epithermal neutron	D_γ/Φ_{epi} (Gy·cm^2/n)	$<2.0 \times 10^{-13}$
Ratio between thermal flux and epithermal flux	Φ_{th}/Φ_{epi}	<0.05
Ratio between neutron current and neutron flux	J/Φ_{epi}	>0.7

delivered to the target treatment volume of the tumor. According to the International Atomic Energy Agency (IAEA)'s recommendation, the intensity of the neutron source must be strong enough to keep the treatment time in under one hour, preferably not more than 30 minutes [1]. Generally, neutrons are classified according to their energy as thermal (E < 0.5 eV), epithermal (0.5 eV < E < 10 keV), and fast (E > 10 keV) neutrons in the context of BNCT. Table 5.2 shows the IAEA's recommendation on beam characteristics of the neutron sources for BNCT. For a detailed description of each parameter, see Section 5.3.2.

5.2.1 *History*

The first generation of neutron sources is radioisotope sources based on natural α radiation. As previously mentioned, Chadwick identified neutrons for the first time in 1932 by using the interaction of α particles from decay of natural polonium with beryllium [3,4]. Subsequently, M. Goldhaber helped Chadwick in discovering the capture of slow neutrons by lithium and boron nuclei in 1934 [5–7]. He also found that the slow neutron disintegration of nitrogen yields an energetic proton in 1936 [8,9].

$$^{10}B + {}^1n \rightarrow {}^7Li + {}^4He$$
$$^6Li + {}^1n \rightarrow {}^4He + {}^3H$$
$$^{14}N + {}^1n \rightarrow {}^{14}C + {}^1H$$

That year, although G. L. Locher proposed neutron capture therapy, he never implemented a slow-neutron-capture experiment [10]. The first attempt, transferred to Crocker Radiation Laboratory on the UC Berkeley campus afterwards due to the intensity of neutrons, was made on the world's second cyclotron that furnished an external ion beam at University of Illinois in 1938 by P. G. Kruger, Goldhaber and B.V. Hall [11].

In the early stages of BNCT, clinical research was carried out almost exclusively with reactor-based neutron sources. It was initiated in 1951 by William H. Sweet [12,13], as well as Lee E. Farr *et al.* at the Brookhaven Graphite Research Reactor and Massachusetts General Hospital (MGH), where borax-mediated BNCT for glioblastoma (GBM) patients transported from Boston to Brookhaven National Laboratory (BNL) was implemented [14–16]. Thereafter, events shifted to the Brookhaven Medical Research Reactor (BMRR) and Massachusetts Institute of Technology Research Reactor (MITR), as the reactors there, designed and constructed specifically for thermal neutron NCT, were aimed at higher flux neutron beams that shorten the irradiation time. However, the outcomes of BNCT trials during 1959–1961 in both BNL and MIT were not satisfactory as had been anticipated, with average survival times less than six months, which resulted in suspension of clinical trials of BNCT in the U.S. [17,18]. Despite all this, the physicist and technician Ralph H. Fairchild in BNL launched an epithermal neutron converter program in 1962 [19], which finally achieved utility in the 1990s [20,21].

In the 1960s, boron compounds that would enter glioma tissues but not cross the blood-brain barrier were first synthesized [22,23] and applied to BNCT studies initially at the MGH [24]. In August 1968, Hiroshi Hatanaka started a clinical trial of BNCT irradiation in Japan, using disodium mercaptoundecahydro-*closo*-dodecaborate, *i.e.*, $Na_2B_{12}H_{11}SH$ (BSH), as the boron compound [25]. He reported exciting results that 49 patients were treated with BNCT at the Hitachi Training Reactor (1968–1975) and Musashi Institute of Technology Research Reactor (1975–1989) until March 1989 [26], and the 5-year survival rate was 58% in a small group of highly selected patients suffering from grade III–IV gliomas. However, these were performed as intraoperative irradiation to increase penetration of the thermal neutron beam. Although the results were favorable, Hatanaka was unable to convince neurosurgeons and radiation oncologists of the usefulness of BNCT. On the bright side, this led to a reconsideration of clinical research with BNCT in the U.S. as well as in Europe.

Hatanaka and his group treated patients with malignant brain tumors, using BSH and thermal neutron beam at five reactors. Besides the two mentioned above, the other three were Japan Research Reactor-3 (JRR3) (1969), JRR2 (1990–1995), and Research Reactor Institute of Kyoto University (KUR, 1974 and 1990–1995) [27]. In 1987, Mishima started a new BNCT trial for malignant melanoma patients using p-boronophenylalanine (BPA) at KUR [28,29]. Furthermore, in February 1994 BPA was first used in BNCT to treat a patient with recurrent malignant glioma at KUR. From 1995 to 1996, KUR was remodeled and neutron energy spectra from thermal to epithermal became available [30]. As of Nov 2014, 510 clinical irradiations were carried out using the KUR facility [31]. Another reactor of JAERI, JRR-4, started clinical trials in 1998, and provided the epithermal neutron beam from 1999. However, in December 2007, a crack in a graphite reflector of the reactor core was found on a weld of the aluminum cladding. JRR-4 was stopped until February 2010 for replacement of the graphite reflector. After restarting BNCT in 2010, three patients were treated. Because of the March 2011 East Japan earthquake and tsunami, JRR-4 was stopped again with no prospect of restarting [32]. In total 107 patients had been treated at JRR-4 [33].

As mentioned above, after the epithermal neutron beam became available at BNL and MIT in the 1990s, the clinical trial with BPA was soon conducted for GBM patients at BMRR (1994–1998) [34] and MITR (1996–1999) [35]. The emergence of BNCT in Europe soon appeared at Petten, the Netherlands [36], then in Finland [37], Sweden [38], the Czech Republic [39] and later in Argentina [40], Taiwan [41] and China [42]. The first clinical trial of BNCT in Europe for the treatment of GBM was carried out in July 1997 at the High Flux Reactor (HFR) in Petten, which was owned by the European Commission [1]. In Finland, the BNCT facility FiR 1 was modified during the 1990s at Espoo [37], and an open phase I BNCT study on GBM was initiated in May 1999 [43]. Before the FiR 1 decommissioning in 2012, more than 200 patients were treated with BNCT for GBM and head & neck tumor [44]. The construction of BNCT facility THOR (Tsing Hua Open-pool Reactor) in Taiwan started in 2000 and finished in 2005. The clinical trials launched until August 2010, treating 26 patients in two different protocols (17+9). In 2017, this facility received the emergent (compassionate) treatment approval from the Taiwan Food and Drug Administration, and continued actively accumulating cases as of 2019 [45]. The nuclear reactors used for BNCT, which are limited, highly expensive and not located in a hospital environment, are either no longer open, have stopped their BNCT programs, or are under the threat of closure. As a promising treatment modality, BNCT did not happen in a hospital environment, which was a barrier to its development [46]. One possible alternative is the use of accelerators to generate enough neutron flux.

Although the first BNCT attempt used a cyclotron as the neutron beam generator, reactor neutron source had been the only choice of BNCT for a long period. With advances in accelerator and neutron science, hospital-based neutron sources for BNCT is now starting to be realized with the support of local policies and finances. The development of accelerator-based neutron sources (ABNS) began in the U.S. in the 1980s, and in 1994 an international workshop sponsored by the U.S. Department of Energy was held [47]. In the next few years, several research groups did in fact successfully design, construct and demonstrate fully functional prototypes for ABNS that were near-clinical in scale, or that demonstrated scalability to clinical levels [48]. However, since the federal funding reduced near 2000, significant advances were made in other parts of the world [49]. The different types of ABNS for BNCT have been reviewed in detail by Nigg [48] and Kreiner [50–52]. Japan is by far the country devoting the largest effort to this endeavor. In Japan, after years of effort since 2008 [53], the world's first treatment system using a combination of a cyclotron and a beryllium target has received manufacturing and marketing approval as a medical device in 2020 [54]. Two facilities that assembled this system for clinical use are Southern Tohoku BNCT Research Center (Fukushima, Japan) and Kansai BNCT Medical Center (Osaka Medical College, Osaka, Japan).

In Tokyo, a different system using a linac (short for linear accelerator) and a lithium target was installed at National Cancer Center (NCC) Hospital, where a phase I clinical trial of BNCT for malignant melanoma and angiosarcoma is underway. Presently, besides Japan, Finland [55], UK, Russia, Argentina, Israel, Italy, USA, China and more recently the Republic of Korea and Spain [56] are actively engaged in the development of ABNS.

5.2.2 Reactor-Based Neutron Sources

The performance characteristics of reactor-based neutron sources have been summarized by Harling and Riley [57], and the suggestion for epithermal neutron irradiation facilities, suitable for high throughput, routine clinical BNCT is discussed by Harling [58]. The earliest BNCT research employed low-energy thermal neutrons because it is relatively easy to create by a fission reactor and the unwanted fast neutron and γ ray contamination are virtually negligible. However, the inadequate useful penetration of the thermal neutron beams (3–4 cm) was soon found in the earliest clinical trials at BNL and MIT, in which intraoperative irradiation was used by Sweet to increase neutron penetration for treatment of GBM, and this approach was subsequently continued in Japan by Hatanaka. With more energetic neutrons, epithermal neutron beams can be moderated in tissues to produce improved thermal neutron distributions at significantly greater depths, which could be used to treat deep-seated tumors (approximately 8 cm deep) without the need to surgically open the cranium.

Two approaches have been used for the design of epithermal neutron irradiation facilities at fission reactors. The most common approach is to use the reactor core directly, attributed to the rapidly growing interest in BNCT of a significant number of research reactors since the 1990s. The modification consisted of removing as much moderator as possible on one core face and adding a large area beam line with filter moderators, thermal neutron and photon shielding and some collimation [59]. With this approach, reactors ranging between 100 kW and several MW were converted successfully, located mainly in the U.S., Europe and Asia. As mentioned above, ten or more facilities such as the low-power (250 kW) Finnish TRIGA (Training, Research, Isotopes, General, Atomics) reactor FiR 1, the 5 MW KUR and 3.5 MW JRR-4 in Japan, and the high-power (45 MW) reactor HFR at Petten have been constructed for clinical use.

A second approach to modifying existing reactors is to use a subcritical array of fuel called a fission converter, originally proposed by Rief *et al.* [60], that is located outside the reactor core and produces fission neutrons from thermalized neutrons emanating from the reactor. The first such facility, known as the fission converter beam (FCB), was constructed at the 5 MW MITR [61]. A few other similar facilities have been designed, such as the 3 MW BMRR [62] and the 2 MW McClellan Air Force Base Reactor [63]. This particular design is appropriate for higher power or multipurpose research reactors without a movable core that support a broad range of experiments.

Whether using the reactor core directly or a fission converter, careful initial design consideration of reactor beams for BNCT should generally result in better and less expensive facilities than those made by retrofitting existing reactors. In 2009, a miniature (30 kW) neutron source reactor called INHI designed for BNCT was constructed near a hospital site in Beijing, China [64]. This is the first reactor constructed specifically for BNCT since the 1950s, based on an ultra-safe, low-cost design. Table 5.3 lists the important parameters of a number of BNCT facilities that have been designed and installed around the world [65].

From the engineering and physical viewpoint, the general requirements of a reactor-based BNCT facility contains the components shown in Figure 5.7 [65]:

(1) *The Reactor*
Over the years, a wide variety of reactors have been used as the neutron source for BNCT. Some of them have been mentioned above, while more facilities were recently reported to participate such as in Poland, Germany, Bulgaria and Iran [66].

(2) *The Beam Tube*
In most cases, an epithermal neutron beam is suggested to be the most ideal beam because it has the greatest potential to treat many tumor

Table 5.3   Beam characteristics for reactor-based BNCT facilities around the world.

	Epithermal Neutron Contamination (109 n/cm²s)	Photon Contaminati on (10^{-13} Gy·cm²)	Fast Neutron Contamination (10^{-13} Gy·cm²)	Beam Diameter (cm)	Positioning Angle (°)	Medical Room Area (m²)
MIT w/o FCB, filter	6.4[a]	3.6	1.4	12	180	14
USA Li filter	3.0[a]	4.6	2.3			
Studsvik, Sweden	1.4	12.6	8.3	14 × 10	180	—
FiR-1, Finland	1.2	0.9	3.3	14	<180	6.4
BMRR, USA	1.1	1.5	2.6	12	180	20
Rez, Czech Republic	0.6	10.8	16.9	12	<180	8.8
HFR EC, NL	0.33	3.8	12.1	12	180	12.2
JRR-4, Japan	2.2	2.6	3.1	12	<180	7.8
KUR, Japan	0.46	2.8	6.2	15	<180	27
THOR, Taiwan	1.7	1.3	2.8	14	180	20

[a]Modified according to [57].

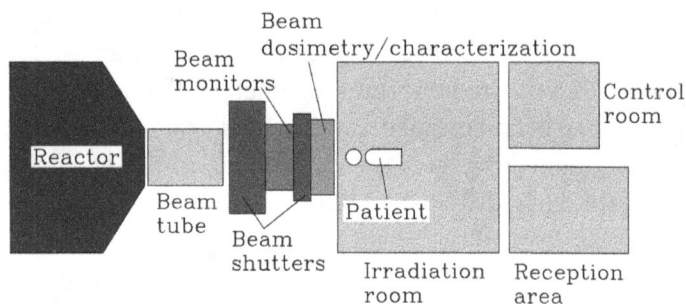

Figure 5.7   General requirements of a reactor-based BNCT facility.

types, especially deep tumors. The quality of epithermal neutron beams for BNCT requires necessary tradeoffs between beam intensity and purity from unwanted photons and neutrons. Neutron and γ beams from the reactor need to be moderated, filtered and attenuated so that the desired beam intensity and average neutron energy are within the required ranges. The neutron beam parameters in Table 5.2 are recommended.

(3) *The Patient*
The type of tumor to be treated by BNCT may influence the beam design, such as the tumor site, angle and depth for beam to irradiate. Whether the patient can only be treated in a horizontal or seated position should also be taken into consideration.

(4) *The Irradiation Room*
For safety reasons, the shielding of the irradiation room and other treatment-related areas should be the priority. Sufficient space for treatment is also essential. The design of a medical irradiation room is paramount in alleviating the limitations inherent in a fixed beamline by providing sufficient space to accommodate staff and equipment, as well as the flexibility to orient the patient in any direction for fields on any part of the body. The room itself should contain most facilities expected in a conventional radiotherapy room, *e.g.*, cameras, laser positioning devices, ease-of-access, *etc.* In some facilities, a pre-positioning area outside the irradiation room is available to shorten the positioning time and help reassure the patient.

(5) *The Control or Observation Room*
The patient and the facility need to be monitored. Monitoring equipment such as pulse oximeters, TV monitors, microphones, radiation level instruments, radiation monitors measuring the beam characteristics, *etc.*, all need to be placed in this room, where the medical and physics personnel can sit comfortably and observe the patient and radiation beam parameters. It should be situated next to the irradiation room.

(6) *Reception Area*
An area should be available where the patient can be received prior to treatment. The preparation of the patient, such as drug infusion, clothes changing, and medical examination is necessary. This area should also include an office for the medical staff, and a waiting area for the relatives of patients.

(7) *The Beam Monitors*
The beam monitoring system, that controls the stability of the beam during the treatment, must be able to measure the radiation beam

during the irradiations and have the capacity to automatically cut off the beam or shut down the beam irradiation system when the required dose is achieved or when an emergency situation occurs. As with conventional radiotherapy, all safety systems should have a back-up system in case of failure. In BNCT, a beam monitoring system normally consists of paired neutron counters and γ ray counters, which are located close to the beam line, usually in the wall of the beam tube or in the collimator, downstream from any beam shutter.

(8) *Beam Shutters*
According to the design of the reactor, the setting of the beam shutter varies with the reactor type, reactor power, and space limitation. The general requirement is to be able to stop or reduce, on demand, radiation levels to a level where staff can enter the irradiation room. For reactors such as the FiR-1 in Finland which have a short beamline without much space for beam control shutters, beam output is controlled by manipulating reactor power. At multipurpose facilities such as HFR and MITR, the reactor operates continuously for long periods of time to service various experimental needs, and it is not feasible to alter reactor power except in emergency situations. Hence, these facilities employ a series of beamline shutters to switch the beam on and off, allowing free access to the medical room even when the reactor is at full power. Beam shutters are generally made of layers of lead and borated or lithiated polyethylene, and usually equipped with an interlock system to enable automatic shutdown when the required dose is achieved and to achieve remotely opening and closing the beam. In case of emergency, manual mode is also available.

(9) *Beam Dosimetry/Characterization*
The radiation beam is a mixture of neutrons, of all energy ranges, and γ rays. Whether as part of a quality assurance system, or as a need for calculations adjustment in treatment planning, the beam must be fully characterized. There are a variety of techniques available to characterize the radiation beam [67].

5.2.3 Accelerator-Based Neutron Sources

The advancement of BNCT requires neutron sources suitable for installation in hospital environments. Low-power accelerators are the most appropriate solution for this purpose. The accelerator offers potential advantages over reactor-based neutron sources for clinical applications. First, neutron fields can be turned on or off as required. Although the target disposal is still an issue to be addressed, there are no issues such as nuclear waste disposal of nuclear reactors, which means that it is possible to apply for medical devices-related licensing and regulation. Second, accelerators have been a prominent feature of radiotherapy departments in hospitals for years, and as a result, clinicians have a long history of using similar devices to perform radiation therapy on patients. Third, the spectrum of neutrons from spallation is much "softer" (lower energy) than that from fission, which makes it easier to produce the "ideal" epithermal neutron spectrum needed to treat a deep-seated tumor, and thus the quality of the neutron field can be designed to significantly exceed the quality of that for a reactor-based neutron source.

An ABNS for BNCT consists of: (1) the accelerator hardware for generating high-current charged particle beams, (2) an appropriate neutron-generating target and target heat removal system, and (3) a beam shaping assembly (*i.e.*, a moderator/reflector assembly) enabling the flux energy spectrum of neutrons produced in the target to be suitable for patient irradiation. There are many different types of accelerators ranging from low-energy electrostatic machines to higher-energy cyclotrons and to much higher-energy linacs or synchrotrons, which have been considered as neutron sources for BNCT. The clinical requirements for neutron field quality and intensity determine the particle reactions that occur in the target, as well as the design and performance requirements of the accelerator. Lithium and beryllium are often used as target materials; they have different properties such as physical properties, neutron yield, neutron energy, thermal neutron properties and activation on proton irradiation in terms of the maintenance of a target. The performance requirements of accelerators targeting Be are more demanding than those of Li target. On the other hand, the low melting point of Li requires a strong target heat load removal ability. Recognizing this trade-off allows physicists and engineers to decide where they want to strike that balance.

An accelerator propels charged particles, such as protons or electrons, at high speeds, close to the speed of light. Accelerators are usually classified as linear or circular accelerator. Below we only discuss the BNCT facilities based on proton accelerators, in which protons are accelerated and transported to a target, where they collide to generate neutrons through nuclear reactions.

5.2.3.1 Cyclotrons

A cyclotron is an example of a circular accelerator (Figure 5.8), which was firstly built by Lawrence and his students in 1931 [68]. Accelerators use electromagnetic fields to accelerate and steer particles. Radiofrequency cavities boost the particle beams, while magnets focus the beams and bend their trajectory. In a cyclotron, the particles repeat the same accelerating path for as long as necessary, gaining an energy boost at each turn, until achieving the desired energy and being extracted. In theory,

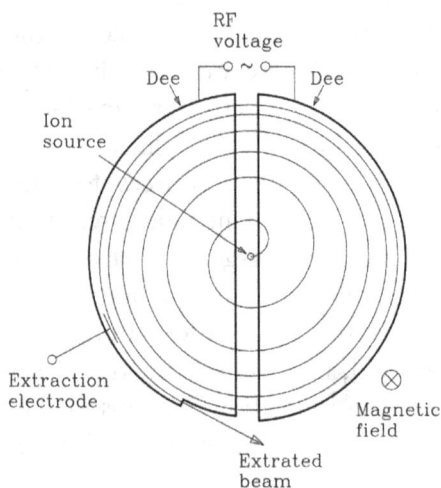

Figure 5.8 A classical cyclotron in plan view. Reproduced with permission from https://cds.cern.ch/record/1513944/files/CERN-2013-001-p17.pdf.

the energy could be increased over and over again. However, the more energy the particles have, the stronger the magnetic fields have to be to keep them in circular orbits. Cyclotrons can be very compact, efficient and cost effective, while the disadvantages are the generally limited lower beam currents compared to linear accelerators. Also, the magnet systems can be large, expensive, and power consuming, and particle extraction can be difficult.

Cyclotrons are now commonly used in hospital settings as positron emitters, which require charged particle beams of higher energy, but significantly less current, than beams that are thought to be optimum for an ABNS for BNCT. Thus, cyclotrons are unlikely candidates for accelerator-based BNCT. However, in Japan, Tanaka *et al.* reported the installation of a 1 mA, 30 MeV proton cyclotron combined with a Be target at KUR in 2008, planned as an alternative to the reactor KUR-HWNIF [53,69]. Medical dosimetry comparation between accelerator-based and reactor-based BNCT [70] as well as beam dosimetry results were reported thereafter [71]. In 2012, the world's first phase I clinical trial using cyclotron BNCT for recurrent malignant glioma in collaboration with Osaka Medical and Pharmaceutical University started, which was conducted in combination with a boron drug manufactured by Stella Pharma Co. Ltd. And in 2014, a phase I clinical trial for head and neck cancer was started in collaboration with Kawasaki Medical School. From the same year, this system started to be established at the Southern Tohoku BNCT Research Center, as a post-earthquake revitalization project, supported by the local government of Fukushima [72]. The phase II clinical trials for recurrent malignant glioma at this facility began in 2016, and phase II head and neck cancer clinical trials also started from that year [73]. Based on the results, Sumitomo Heavy Industries Ltd. together with Stella Pharma Co. Ltd applied for BNCT approval in October 2019, and in March 2020 received approval from the Japanese Ministry of Health, Labor and Welfare for the manufacture and sale of medical devices (BNCT system "NeuCure® System" and dose calculation program "NeuCure® Dose Engine") and pharmaceuticals (Steboronine®). The approved indication is unresectable locally advanced or locally recurrent head and neck cancer. More indications such as recurrent malignant gliomas are pending approval [74].

Table 5.4   Main specifications of HM-30 cyclotron.

Particle	Negative hydrogen ion	Extraction method	Foil stripping
Injection energy	30 keV	Extraction energy	30 MeV
Injection method	Axial injection	Extracted maximum beam current	2 mA
RF frequency	73.1 MHz	Nominal operation current	1 mA
RF accelerating voltage	200 kV/turn	Magnet size	W3.0m × D1.6m × H1.7m
Harmonic number	4	Weight	60 tons

The cyclotron named HM-30 accelerates H⁻ to 30 MeV, and proton beam is extracted by a carbon foil stripper. Main specifications are listed in Table 5.4 [75].

At the proton energy region from several MeV to ~200 MeV, an AVF cyclotron is small and cost effective compared to other accelerators. AVF is an abbreviation for "Azimuthally Varying Field." It means that the strength of the magnetic field varies in the azimuthal (beam path) direction in order to converge the beam in radial and axial directions, which was proposed by Thomas in 1938. Variations can be added to the confinement magnetic field by attaching wedge-shaped inserts at periodic azimuthal positions of the magnet poles. The additional horizontal field components enhance vertical focusing. Average negative field index can be tolerated so that the bending field increases with radius. With proper choice of focusing elements and field index variation, the magnetic field variation balances the relativistic mass increase, resulting in a constant revolution frequency. AVF cyclotrons with this property are called isochronous cyclotrons. Another advantage of AVF cyclotrons is that the stronger vertical focusing allows higher beam intensity. The original thought of AVF cyclotrons is shown in Figure 5.9.

In order to realize 30 MeV and mA-order proton beam acceleration, the following techniques are adopted for HM-30. First, negative hydrogen ion acceleration and foil stripping extraction are realized. A proton beam of 30 MeV and 2 mA means a beam power of 60 kW.

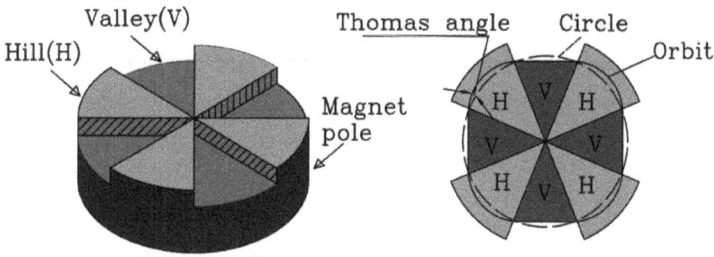

Figure 5.9 Magnetic fields in an AVF cyclotron (left) and non-circular shape of orbit (right). Reproduced with permission from Pearson, E., Kleeven, W., Nuttens, V., *et al.* (2016). Development of Cyclotrons for Proton and Particle Therapy. In: Rath, A. K. and Sahoo, N. (Eds.), *Particle Radiotherapy: Emerging Technology for Treatment of Cancer*, Springer, pp. 21–36.

In the case of positive ion acceleration, beam loss at the electrical deflector is unavoidable. It causes localized heating or additional sources of radiation to limit the beam current. In the case of acceleration of negative ions, they change to positive ions through a thin foil placed on the extraction orbit. Due to the opposite curvature of the positive ions in the magnet, almost 100% of the positive ions are automatically extracted from the accelerating orbit. This method can handle high-power beams without losses. Secondly, high-current external ion source and vertical injection are used. A multi-cusp ion source provides a beam of negative hydrogen ions more than 10 mA, injected vertically into the cyclotron. This vertical line consists of a focusing solenoid, a buncher, and a spiral inflector. The spiral inflector is carefully optimized for high-current beams. Although the facility employs a cyclotron having to deal with a very hard neutron spectrum and hence with a very high activation, it is still a big step toward an in-hospital BNCT facility.

5.2.3.2 *Linear Accelerators*

In contrast to circular accelerator, a linear accelerator is exclusively formed of accelerating structures since the particles do not need to be deflected, but they only benefit from a single acceleration pass. Linear accelerators can be classified as electrostatic linear accelerators or RF (radiofrequency) linear accelerators. As the name suggests, in an electrostatic linear accelerator, charged particles are accelerated by an electrostatic field. In contrast, in a RF linear accelerator, charged particles are accelerated by a time-varying induced electric field.

5.2.3.2.1 Electrostatic linear accelerators

Using high-voltage terminals that keep a static potential of around a few millions volts, charged particles can be accelerated. In simple terms, an electrostatic generator is basically a giant capacitor. In the earliest days when accelerators were built, the high voltage is achieved either using the methods of Van de Graaff proposed in 1929 or Cockcroft & Walton in 1932 [68]. In a Van de Graaff accelerator, the accelerating potential is generated by physically transporting charge on a moving sheet or belt to an upper terminal where it was removed. The terminal was in the form of a large sphere, the shape that best holds charge without creating a spark. This voltage was then applied (as in Cockcroft-Walton machines) to an accelerating column down which particles accelerated from high voltage to ground. The maximum energy of particles in such accelerators is practically limited by the discharge limit of the high-voltage platform, which is about 12 MV at ambient atmospheric conditions. Typically, this limit is increased by housing the high-voltage platform in an insulating gas tank with a dielectric constant above air, such as SF_6 (sulfur hexafluoride, 2.5 times the dielectric constant of air), which is chemically inert and non-toxic, increasing the maximum voltage up to around 30 MV and minimizing sparking. To increase the maximum acceleration energy further, the tandem concept was invented to use the same high voltage twice (Figure 5.10), which means that negative ions

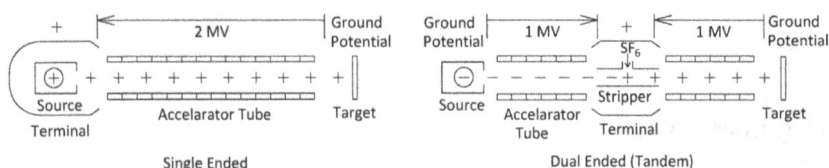

Figure 5.10 Schematic of single-ended DC (left) and tandem or dual ended (right). Reproduced with permission from https://www.pelletron.com/products/tandem-vs-single-ended/.

are accelerated from the ion source (which is held at ground potential) to a stripping foil (which is held at positive potential). At the stripping foil, the accelerated negative ions are stripped of their electrons, leaving positively charged ions, which are further accelerated to the target, as like the source, remaining at ground potential.

(1) *Single-ended DC*
A single-ended DC linear accelerator for the generation of high-current, high-energy ion beams which can be used in BNCT generally includes an ion source for the creation of the ion beam, an analyzing magnet to purify the ion beam, an accelerating tube, a DC high-voltage power supply and a separate pumping tube that transports the vast majority of the neutral gas from the ion source at high voltage toward a vacuum pump at ground potential, thereby preventing the adverse influence of increased vacuum pressure inside the accelerating tube to facilitate stable acceleration of high-current beams to high energies. At the present time, a large number of high-current single-ended DC linear accelerators have diverse purposes and are applied to a wide range of scientific and industrial tasks, such as cyclotron injection, ion beam analysis of materials, accelerator mass spectroscopy, silicon cleaving, ion implantation in semiconductor devices, ion beam cancer therapy, *etc.*, because the accelerators can be used to accelerate particles of various charges and masses to various energies.

The nuBeam® manufactured by Neutron Therapeutics Inc. (NTI, Danvers, MA, USA) is one of such electrostatic accelerators, formerly known as Hyperion, a single-ended electrostatic accelerator designed to operate at 40–50 mA and 2.0 MeV. For a BNCT clinic built at the Helsinki University Hospital, NTI manufactured a nuBeam® system with 2.6 MeV, 30 mA single-ended DC electrostatic accelerator with a rotating lithium target, which is under commissioning [55]. Clinical trials with patients of inoperable, locally recurrent head and neck cancer will be initiated if the Finnish Radiation and Nuclear Safety Authority gives approval. NTI has also agreed with the Tokushukai Medical Group to install a nuBeam® system for BNCT at Shonan Kamakura General Hospital in Kamakura, Japan. And recently High-Flux Accelerator-Driven Neutron Facility (HHUF, Birmingham, UK) and Institut Jules Bordet (IJB, University Hospital of Brussels, Brussels,

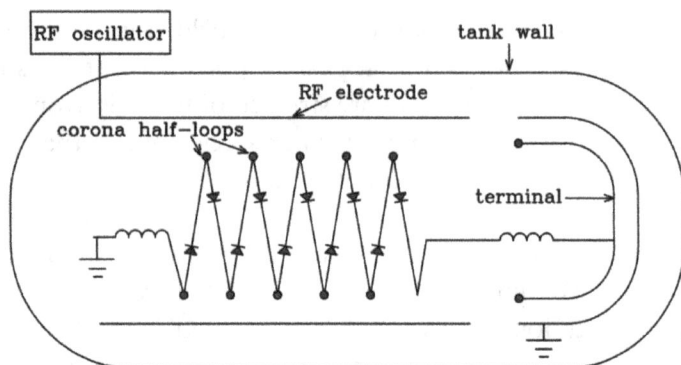

Figure 5.11 Schematic of the Dynamitron. Reproduced with permission from http://capturedlightning.com/Papers/DC-accel-DB1.pdf.

Belgium) announced the installation of this system for neutron science research and BNCT clinical use, respectively.

(2) Dynamitron

The Dynamitron has been developed by Radiation Dynamics, Inc. (RDI, Long Island, USA) since 1958, initially designed for the acceleration of high-intensity electron beams (Figure 5.11). The source can be changed to accelerate other types of particles. It is a single-ended machine enclosed in an SF_6-filled pressurized vessel, and the high voltage is generated through rectified RF power. A Cockcroft-Walton-like cascade generator provides the DC voltage. In modern machines, semiconductor diodes are used. RF chokes provide the connection of the rectifier cascade between ground and high voltage terminal. A rectifier stage consists of two rectifier diodes. Due to the absence of moving parts inside the pressure vessel, the advantage of this power supply is high reliability. Another advantage compared to the classical Cockcroft-Walton generator is the very low capacitance of the system. Therefore, possible sparks are virtually harmless. The regulation loop of a Dynamitron generator can be modeled like a standard electronic power supply. As a result, the terminal voltage stabilizes significantly faster than a classical Van de Graaff belt generator.

There was a proposal to establish a BNCT facility with an existing Dynamitron accelerator at the University of Birmingham, UK in 1995 [76]. This linear electrostatic accelerator was initially operated with the capability of producing beam currents of up to 1 mA of 2.5–3.0 MeV protons, and later upgraded to 5 mA in 1998 [77]. With the constrains on beam current and beam orientation (the beam is directed vertically downward), research started to explore further the design options available in moving toward a clinical facility, in particular, to look at the feasibility of using a horizontally extracted neutron therapy beam with a vertical proton beam. It was concluded that a proton beam energy of 2.8 MeV incident on a lithium target is optimum. In order to conduct an optimal clinical program, this machine would need an upgrade in terms of beam current, a goal of which was initially 10 mA, and increased to 20 mA in 2009, proposed by Ion Beam Applications (IBA, Louvain-la-Neuve, Belgium) [78]. With an upgraded electron cyclotron resonance (ECR) ion source, beam currents above 35 mA of 30 keV protons and molecular hydrogen have been measured at source exit of the machine. A permanent magnet filtered out molecular hydrogen to select protons and injected them in the accelerator. The accelerating voltage range is from 1.9 to 2.8 MV.

The Industry-Academia Joint Laboratory was established at Nagoya University, Japan in 2013 to develop an ABNS for BNCT [79]. The facility named Nagoya University Accelerator-driven Neutron Source (NUANS) installed an IBA-manufactured Dynamitron, supplying high current proton beam with 2.8 MeV proton energy and 15 mA DC beam current, and feasibility studies on neutron production for the BNCT will be launched after the commissioning. The maximum beam power is 42 kW. The overall dimensions are 7.5 m × 2.8 m and the weight is 8.5 tons. Two beamlines were planned to be installed. For the time being, the neutron source for BNCT is installed at the end of the first beamline. The aim of this neutron source is as an evaluation test machine of Li target for BNCT. There are plans to install a second beamline for scientific and engineering experiments. The NUANS has been used to generate neutrons as part of the facility commissioning since 2018 [80].

(3) *Tandem*

It was reported in 1997 that an electrostatic accelerator was installed for BNCT research at MIT [81]. The accelerator was built in a tandem configuration that produced beam currents exceeding 1 mA at a voltage of 2 MV (4 MeV proton and deuteron beams) [82]. The high beam current was achieved through improving the lifetime of stripping foil (a carousel containing 82 foils that can be moved into place) and placing tiny permanent magnets on accelerating electrodes to avoid the electrostatic breakdown exacerbated by counter-streaming electrons (electrons that travel in the opposite direction as the protons in the beam). An active research program, including animal studies aimed at developing BNC synovectomy, unfolded around that machine.

Another facility has been built based on a vacuum-insulated compact tandem accelerator (VITA) at the Budker Institute of Nuclear Physics (BINP) in Novosibirsk, Russia, proposed since 1998 [83]. It is intended to generate neutrons with the threshold $^7Li(p, n)^7Be$ reaction by bombarding a lithium target with a 2–2.5 MeV, 10 mA proton beam. The first accelerated protons were obtained in 2008. To date, the maximum currents achieved are at about 9 mA [84]. Numerous improvements to achieve the stable tandem work and to increase the accelerated proton beam current have been made over the years. Milestones include the first significant increase in proton beam current to 5 mA in 2015, which was achieved after the suppression of secondary electrons produced by accelerated argon ions flowing from the gas target and ionized by the beam. The upgrade also improved the operational stability of the accelerator. And the DC Penning negative ion source was upgraded several times to increase output beam current as well, such as the latest improvement of introducing differential pumping system equipped with two high-performance turbomolecular pumps with pumping speed of 2,200 l/s, which permitted an increased DC H⁻ beam output of 10 mA. The VITA system is now undergoing further upgrades. And the clinical project of the system has been launched in Xiamen Humanity Hospital (Xiamen, Fujian, China). A 2.5 MeV, 10 mA new system was manufactured and installed by Neuboron Medtech Ltd. (Nanjing, Jiangsu, China), TAE Life Sciences (Foothill Ranch, CA, USA), and BINP [85]. Commissioning of the new facility has been completed, and is about to enter the clinical trial phase. In addition, National Center of Oncological Hadrontherapy (CNAO, Pavia, Italy) and Blokhin National Medical Research Center of

Oncology (Moscow, Russia) also announced the system for BNCT clinical applications.

(4) Electrostatic Quadrupole Accelerator
A BNCT project was proposed at Lawrence Berkeley Laboratory (LBNL) in the 1990s to develop a 2.5 MeV, 100 mA proton single-ended electrostatic quadrupole (ESQ) accelerator [86]. In an ESQ system, distances between differently charged structures are increased to mitigate the possibility of electrostatic breakdown, which may enlarge the size of the device. Therefore, the transverse electric field that provides the ESQ focusing is derived from the potentials applied to two pairs of electrodes, which is similar to the magnetic quadrupoles that provides transverse focusing in high-energy accelerators. The advantage of an ESQ system is that the transverse focusing can be very strong (useful for a high-current beam) without incurring a longitudinal field near or exceeding the breakdown limit. Another advantage is that the transverse fields sweep out stray charges generated along the vacuum chamber, thus inhibiting voltage breakdown. The machine at one point in time was refurbished and the main challenge was to develop a suitable power system [87,88].

A project to build an ESQ accelerator facility is under development in Argentina based on the concept developed at LBNL. The group is presently working toward the facility to be installed at the Constituyentes Atomic Center of the Atomic Energy Commission in Buenos Aires, Argentina [89]. The final goal of the project is a machine capable of delivering 30 mA of 1.45 MeV deuterons to be used in conjunction with a neutron production target based on the ^{9}Be(d, n) or ^{13}C(d, n) reaction. In the first stage, the accelerator will be able to produce proton and deuteron beams of about 1.45 MeV [52]. The terminal of the final machine is designed to work in air to facilitate the maintenance and minimize the number of ancillary devices (like a pressure vessel and an SF_6 system). The strong transverse electric quadrupole fields help to keep the beam close to the beam axis, counterbalancing the space charge effects and effectively sweeping ions and electrons created along the acceleration column, hence preventing the generation of discharges along the tubes which contributes to a more stable operation.

5.2.3.2.2 RF linear accelerators

In 1970, Teplyakov and Kapachinskii invented the radiofrequency quadrupole linear accelerator (RFQ) in the Soviet Union, which caught the attention of Western physicists at Los Alamos. RFQ is a low-velocity (range from about 0.01 to 0.06 times the velocity of light), high-current linear accelerator with high capture efficiency that can be used to accelerate any kind of nucleons from a few keV per nucleus up to a few MeV. This is a linear accelerator configuration in which the drift tube has four conducting rods or vanes, placed symmetrically about the beam axis that provides both acceleration and focusing. Strong transverse focusing comes naturally, while the longitudinal components of the electric field, from the radial vane modulations, provide bunching and acceleration of the beam. The schematic of RFQ cavity is shown in Figure 5.12. Acceleration in an RFQ is achieved by periodically modulating the electrodes in the longitudinal direction as shown in Figure 5.13. Because of the very fine periodicity possible in the modulations along the vane (each period corresponding to the effective length of a drift tube), it is particularly useful for low-velocity particles, such as protons and heavy ions. The RFQ bunches and captures the DC beam injected from the ion source, then accelerates the beam to an energy high enough for injection into the drift-tube linac (DTL) for conventional high-intensity proton accelerator design. RFQs as

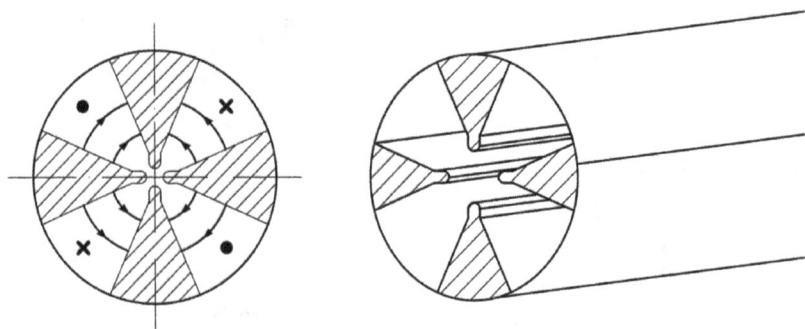

Figure 5.12 Sketch of an RFQ cavity. (Left) The vertically focusing Electric Quad and Magnetic Quad (the ES quad is rotated 45° from the magnetic quad). (Right) The perspective view. Reproduced with permission from Wangler, T. P. (1988). *Principles of RF Linear Accelerators*. John Wiley & Sons.

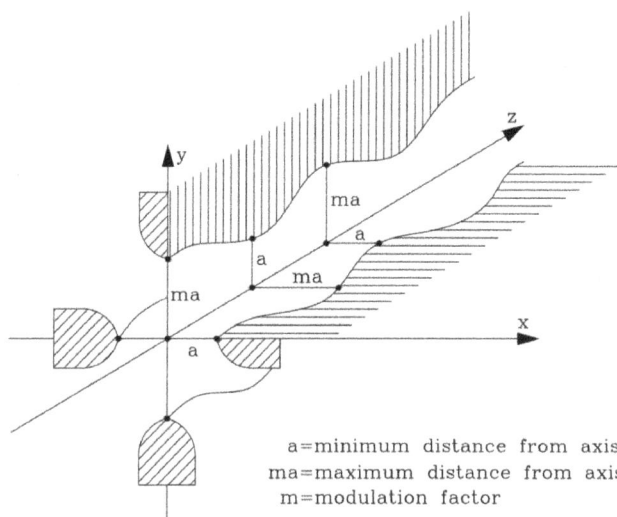

a=minimum distance from axis
ma=maximum distance from axis
m=modulation factor

Figure 5.13 Longitudinal modulation on the RFQ electrodes. Reproduced with permission from Wangler, T. P. (1988). *Principles of RF Linear Accelerators*. John Wiley & Sons.

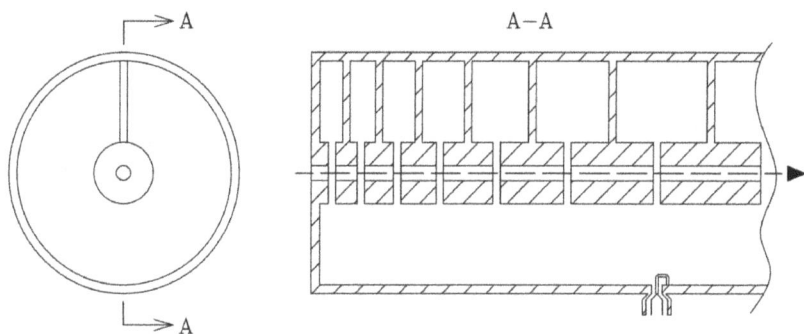

Figure 5.14 Alvarez DTL cavity. Reproduced with permission from Wangler, T. P. (1988). *Principles of RF Linear Accelerators*. John Wiley & Sons.

standalone accelerators also have many applications in ion implantation, isotope production, and neutron sources.

The Alvarez DTL configuration is used for acceleration of protons and other ions in the velocity range from about 0.04 to 0.4 times the speed of light (Figure 5.14). The beam particles are bunched before injection into the DTL, in which the fields in adjacent gaps are in phase, the beam is accelerated in the gap, and the spacing of the accelerating gap is nominally equal to the distance the beam travels in one RF period. When the magnetic fields have the wrong acceleration polarity, they are isolated from the magnetic field by the drift tube. The drift tubes are supported by the stems. The cavity is excited by the RF current flowing into the loop coupler on the coaxial line.

(1) *Standalone RFQ design*
As a candidate for accelerators in BNCT, RF linacs can generate sufficient beam currents for BNCT within limited space constraints, and have great potential for high current operation in order to shorten the treatment time. The RF linac can operate at any duty factor, all the way to 100% duty or a continuous wave (CW) which results in acceleration of beams with high average current. For a CW proton linac (100% duty factor), the peak and average currents are equal, whereas for any pulsed linac, the average current is always less than the peak current. A typical high value for the peak current in a proton linac is about 100 mA, and average currents above about 1 mA are usually considered high values. The main advantage for either CW or longer-pulse operation is to reduce the space-charge forces or other beam current-dependent effects associated with acceleration of beam with high average currents. These effects can be reduced by spreading the total beam charge over more RF buckets, as is done in CW or longer-pulse operation. To shorten the accelerator for a given energy gain, the longitudinal electric field needs to be raised, but this increases the power dissipation and increases the risk of RF electric breakdown. For high-duty-factor operation, the average power density of RF losses on the cavity walls can produce challenging cooling requirements for the conventional copper-cavity technology. RFQs are made of copper, copper-plated mild steel, and aluminum, among other materials. Modern precision machining for monolithic structures with brazing or electroforming in order to obtain the very high precision is required. However, as the beam current increases, the capital and operating costs of the RF power for the accelerator increase. For RF linacs used in BNCT, the choice of RFQ beam current depends on the cost and required treatment time.

A conceptual design of a low-energy neutron generator for treatment of brain tumors by BNCT was proposed in 1989. The concept is based on a 2.5 MeV proton beam from an RFQ linac [90]. The linac was designed for CW operation at a beam current of 30 mA. The extension of the RFQ linac to CW operation is a challenging endeavor. BNCT requires a small and inexpensive RF accelerator that can meet but not greatly exceed the needs for BNCT. Linac Systems LLC (Texas, US) developed a prototype RF linac in 1999 based on a new linac structure that combines an RFQ linac with an RF-focused drift tube (RFD) linac, which was expected to produce a 10 mA, 2.5 MeV proton beam. The RFD linac was designed specifically to increase acceleration efficiency, thereby reducing RF capital and operating costs of linac structures in the few MeV range [91]. Following that, Linac Systems further proposed the RF-focused interdigital linear accelerator structure, which was designed to generate 2.5 MeV protons with an average beam current of 20 mA. The ion source used in this linac is a 2.45 GHz microwave proton source (ECR-type) with a reliable CW mode of operation. It was reported that a design flaw limited the peak current to 12 mA, and attempts have been made to fix it [92].

The Italian National Institute of Nuclear Physics (INFN) designed and constructed an RFQ proton accelerator delivering a 5 MeV, 30 mA proton beam in CW mode [93]. Advantages with respect to high-voltage power supply and CW klystron includes the lower capital and operating costs (cost and duration of components), availability and reliability (non-stop operation in case of component failure), and absence of high voltages (very important for in-hospital operation).

The standalone RFQ design for BNCT was introduced by Cancer Intelligence Care Systems, Inc. (CICS) [94]. By using 2.5 MeV proton beam on lithium target, a high-current (20 mA) beam is required to obtain neutron flux for BNCT. CICS concluded a joint research agreement with NCC (Tokyo, Japan), and an accelerator-based neutron capture therapy device was installed when the hospital's clinical building was completed in 2014. Since then, non-clinical tests have been carried out. The phase I clinical trial aims to evaluate the safety and tolerability of BNCT using the CICS-1 device and the boron compound manufactured by Stella Pharma Co. Ltd., which is designed for patients suffering from malignant melanoma or angiosarcoma, both of which are forms of skin cancer [95].

An experimental facility-based RFQ linac for BNCT research (D-BNCT01) was installed in Dongguan Neutron Science Center

(Dongguan, China). The neutron beam has been successfully produced using a low-current 3.5 MeV proton beam in 2019. Since then, the proton current has gradually increased, and the whole facility has been completed in 2020, which can generate a neutron flux about 1.2×10^8 n/cm^2/s at the beam port using a 5 kW proton beam. The pre-clinical trials have been performed on D-BNCT01. In addition, D-BNCT02, a BNCT facility that will be installed in a hospital, is under construction. D-BNCT02 is planned to generate a proton energy of 2.8 MeV with a beam power of 50 kW [96].

(2) RFQ+DTL Linac

A project team headed by University of Tsukuba, Japan launched the development of a new accelerator-based BNCT facility. In the project, RFQ+DTL linac as proton accelerators have been adopted to manufacture the iBNCT facility. Proton energy generated from the linac was set to 8 MeV and average current was 10 mA. The linac tube has been constructed by Mitsubishi Heavy Industry Co. A building has been renovated for use as BNCT treatment facility in Tokai village. The linac tube had been installed in the facility in September 2012 [97]. The fundamental parameters of the J-PARC were adopted to produce iBNCT linac tubes, so it is possible to utilize the production technology and know-how accumulated during the development of J-PARC. At the same time, the original system was designed and combined with the linac tubes for the peripheral devices of the iBNCT linac, such as ion source, cooling method of the tubes, water cooling system and control system. Construction of the iBNCT was completed at the end of 2015, while neutrons were successfully produced in early 2016 with low-current proton beams. Since then, through the continuous advancement of accelerators, by 2017 the average proton current was increased to more than 1.0 mA. To understand the performance of the device and the physical characteristics of the neutron beam, several experiments have been carried out since mid-2017 [98].

5.2.3.3 Neutron-Generating Targets

In an accelerator-based BNCT facility, neutrons are generated by the nuclear reaction between accelerated protons and a target material. To obtain epithermal neutrons for therapy, the fast neutrons emitting from the target should be moderated to a suitable energy range. In order to reduce the cost and construction difficulty of neutron moderation, the energy of the generated fast neutrons should not be too high.

The ideal target material for BNCT should have the following properties:

(1) Material properties: stable, non-toxic, good thermal conductivity, high melting temperature, low residual radioactivity, no blistering;
(2) The neutron yield is high to shorten the treatment time as much as possible;
(3) The neutron energy spectrum is close to epithermal neutrons, so no moderation is required or the moderation method is simple;
(4) No other radiation, nuclear pollution or radioactive waste will occur in the nuclear reaction that generates neutrons;
(5) The target material is easy to obtain, easy to operate, simple to process, low cost, long service life and easy to maintain.
But in reality, target materials and the corresponding nuclear reactions that meet all the requirements cannot be found on Earth.

Considering the above factors, it is more appropriate to bombard materials of small atomic numbers with lower-energy protons. There are four kinds of nuclear reactions that are relatively close:

(1) $^7Li(p, n)^7Be$

This is an endothermic reaction with the reaction threshold $E_{threshhold}$ = 1.881 MeV, which is quite low. When the incident proton beam energy is in the near-threshold range of 1.91 MeV, the maximum and average energies of the generated neutrons are 105 keV and 42 keV, respectively, which are close to the energy range of epithermal neutrons; the maximum and average emission angles are 60° and 28°, respectively, which ensure the generated neutrons have a high utilization rate.

(2) $^9Be(p, n)^9B$

This is an endothermic reaction with the reaction threshold $E_{threshhold}$ = 2.055 MeV.

(3) ^{9}Be(d, n)^{10}B

This is an exothermic reaction with no reaction threshold. And at relatively low energies, there is also significant neutron production. A dedicated accelerator that accelerates deuterium ions is required to perform this nuclear reaction. A research institution in Argentina has carried out related work in this area, but the current research results are few and this chapter will not describe it in detail.

(4) ^{13}C(d, n)^{14}N

There is no reaction threshold for this nuclear reaction, and the neutron yield is low. There are few related works and applications, which are not discussed here.

Table 5.5 below shows the neutron production rate for each nuclear reaction.

5.2.3.3.1 Properties of Lithium and Beryllium

Lithium is silver-white, soft, and the least dense metal on earth. It is very reactive chemically. At room temperature, it not only can react with water, but also combine with oxygen and nitrogen in the air to

Table 5.5 The neutron production rate for each nuclear reaction.

Reaction	E_{in} (MeV)	Total Production (n/mA s)	Fraction (E_n < 1 MeV)
^{7}Li(p, n)^{7}Be	1.881	0	100%
	1.890	6.3×10^9	100%
	2.300	5.8×10^{11}	100%
	2.500	9.3×10^{11}	100%
	2.800	1.4×10^{12}	92%
^{9}Be(p, n)^{9}B	2.055	0	100%
	2.500	3.9×10^{10}	100%
	4.000	1.0×10^{12}	50%
^{9}Be(d, n)^{10}B	1.450	1.6×10^{11}	69%
	1.500	3.3×10^{11}	50%
^{13}C(d, n)^{14}N	1.500	1.9×10^{11}	70%

Table 5.6   Physical properties of lithium and beryllium.

	Lithium	Beryllium
Relative atomic mass	6.941	9.012
Melting point (°C)	180.54	1,283
Boiling point (°C)	1,342	2,970
Density (g/cm³)	0.534 (25°C) 0.51 (220°C) 0.457 (800°C)	1.847 (25°C)
Specific heat (J/gK)	3.55	1.8828
Thermal conductivity (W/mK)	84.7	201
Heat of fusion (kJ/mol)	3	292.4
Solubility in water	violent reaction occurs to generate a large amount of hydrogen gas	insoluble or slightly soluble

form lithium oxide (Li_2O) and black lithium nitride (Li_3N) crystals. Moreover, it will react with carbon dioxide to form stable lithium carbonate (Li_2CO_3). Therefore, metallic lithium needs to be stored in isolation from air. If it is immersed in kerosene, because of its low density (Table 5.6) it is likely to float on the liquid surface, so it is best to bury it in Vaseline for storage. The melting point of lithium is low, only 180°C.

Beryllium is a light, steel-grey metallic metal. The hardness of beryllium is higher than that of the metals of the same group. Beryllium has the largest heat capacity of all metals. With a specific heat capacity of 1.8828 J/gK at room temperature, beryllium absorbs more heat than other metals, and this property is maintained until its melting point. Beryllium reacts with oxygen at room temperature to form a dense protective film on its surface. Therefore, beryllium is stable even when heated to high temperature in air.

Beryllium compounds such as beryllium oxide, beryllium fluoride, beryllium chloride, beryllium sulfide and beryllium nitrate are relatively toxic, while metal beryllium is less toxic. Beryllium is a systemic poison. The degree of toxicity depends on the route of entry and the physical and chemical properties of different beryllium compounds. Therefore, be careful when handling beryllium and its compounds.

5.2.3.3.2 Neutron Yield of Lithium and Beryllium with Proton

The reaction cross-section data of reaction between protons and lithium/beryllium are obtained from the nuclear database ENDF/B-VIII.0 [2].

It can be seen from Figures 5.15 and 5.16 that the reaction cross-section of lithium and protons is larger than that of beryllium, especially in the low-energy range (proton energy < 6 MeV). If an accelerator with low energy is chosen, it should be matched with a lithium target in order to have higher neutron generation efficiency. Neutrons can be generated in relatively high yields by interacting with lithium using protons with energies just above the reaction threshold. And the energies of the generating neutrons are low, so the desired epithermal neutron beam can be obtained by simple moderation. However, due to the disadvantage of low melting point of lithium mentioned above, if the lithium target is irradiated by a proton beam with energy above about 4 MeV. The target may be subject to a large thermal load, resulting in the risk of lithium melting. Therefore, proton accelerators with energy of 2–4 MeV basically use lithium as the target material, which produces neutrons with high yield, low energy and good forwardness.

The reaction cross-section of beryllium and proton is small, so it is necessary to increase the proton energy (preferably greater than 8 MeV) to increase the neutron yield. The yield, energies and forward directivity of neutrons generated by the reaction vary with the energy of the incident protons. High-energy incident protons will generate high-energy neutrons. If they are to be moderated into epithermal neutrons, there are considerable requirements for the design and construction of the beam shaping assembly.

5.2.3.3.3 Thickness of Target Materials

There is another very important parameter, which is the thickness of the target material. The selection of the thickness of target material is actually related to the distance of protons moving through matter, that is, the range of protons.

When the charged particles move through matter, they constantly lose energy. When the energy is exhausted, they stay in the matter, so

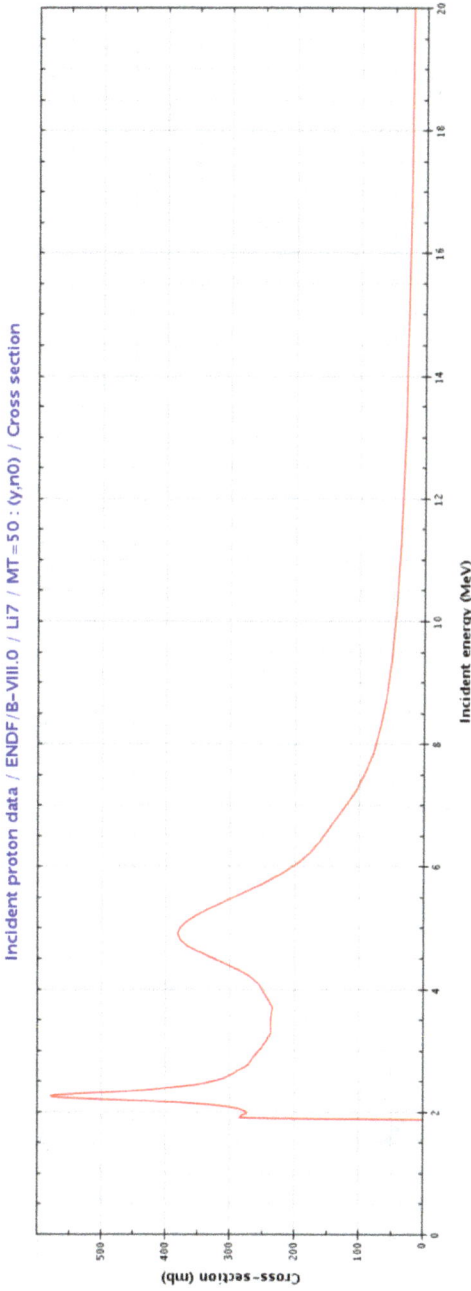

Incident proton data / ENDF/B-VIII.0 / Li7 / MT=50 : (y,n0) / Cross section

Figure 5.15 The cross-section of the reaction between proton and ^{7}Li. The maximum value of the cross-section at about 2.26 MeV is 0.578 barns.

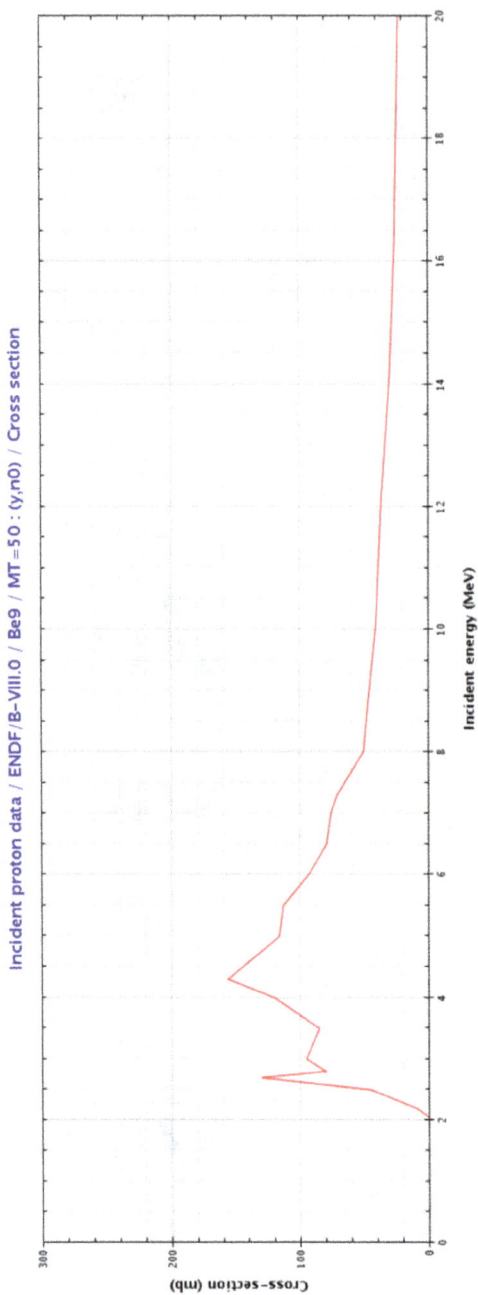

Figure 5.16 The cross-section of the reaction between proton and ^{9}Be. The maximum cross-section at about 4.3 MeV is 0.156 barns.

the particle beam has obvious absorption near the average range. The range (projection range) refers to the straight-line distance of the incident particle from the incident point to its termination point (velocity equals zero) along the incident direction, that is, the depth of penetration along the incident direction.

Because the nuclear reaction (p, n) that produces neutrons has a reaction threshold, the incident proton energy must be greater than the reaction threshold to generate a neutron by nuclear reaction with the target. Therefore, in order to utilize the target material most efficiently, the thickness of the target material should be equal to the range that the protons travel in the target material from the reduction of the incident energy to the reaction threshold (Figure 5.17). If the target material exceeds this thickness, the energy of the proton will drop below the reaction threshold, and the nuclear reaction (p, n) will not occur.

Use SRIM[6] program to calculate the range of protons in order to select the thickness of the target material. The ranges of protons with

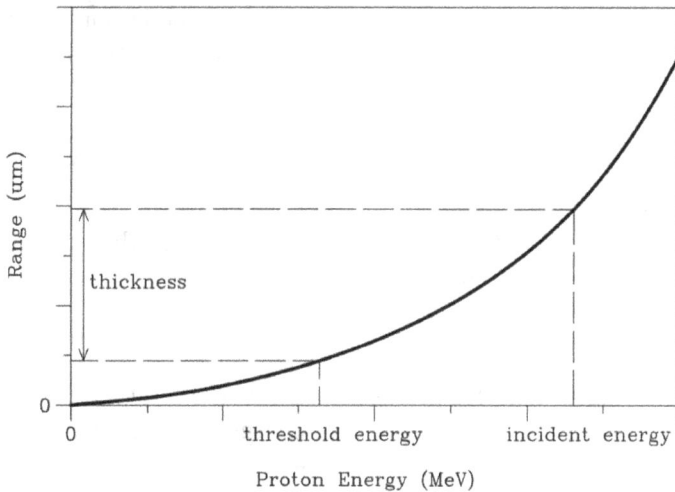

Figure 5.17 Range of protons incident into matter and thickness of target material to be selected.

---

[6]SRIM: The Stopping and Range of Ions in Matter. SRIM is a collection of software packages which calculate many features of the transport of ions in matter. http://www.srim.org/.

```
Ion = Hydrogen [1] , Mass = 1.008 amu

Target Density =  5.3400E-01 g/cm3 = 4.6330E+22 atoms/cm3
======= Target  Composition ========
   Atom    Atom    Atomic    Mass
   Name    Numb    Percent   Percent
   ----    ----    -------   -------
    Li      3      100.00    100.00
=====================================
Bragg Correction = 0.00%
Stopping Units = MeV / (mg/cm2)
See bottom of Table for other Stopping units

     Ion          dE/dx      dE/dx    Projected  Longitudinal  Lateral
    Energy         Elec.      Nuclear    Range     Straggling   Straggling
  ----------     --------   --------  ----------  -----------  ----------
   3.50 MeV     8.918E-02  4.093E-05  418.64 um    16.61 um      8.61 um


Ion = Hydrogen [1] , Mass = 1.008 amu

Target Density =  5.3400E-01 g/cm3 = 4.6330E+22 atoms/cm3
======= Target  Composition ========
   Atom    Atom    Atomic    Mass
   Name    Numb    Percent   Percent
   ----    ----    -------   -------
    Li      3      100.00    100.00
=====================================
Bragg Correction = 0.00%
Stopping Units = MeV / (mg/cm2)
See bottom of Table for other Stopping units

     Ion          dE/dx      dE/dx    Projected  Longitudinal  Lateral
    Energy         Elec.      Nuclear    Range     Straggling   Straggling
  ----------     --------   --------  ----------  -----------  ----------
   1.88 MeV     1.454E-01  7.128E-05  143.25 um     5.02 um      3.15 um
```

Figure 5.18 Range of 3.5 MeV proton when incident on lithium target (upper). Range of 1.881 MeV proton when incident on lithium target (lower).

energies of 3.5 MeV and 1.881 MeV were calculated by SRIM, as shown in Figure 5.18. The subtraction of the two ranges is the thickness (418.64 μm $-$ 143.25 μm ≈ 275 μm) of the lithium that should be selected. Similarly, the thickness of the beryllium target can be selected.

Another advantage of selecting the thickness of the target material in this way is that it can avoid the target from being subjected to too much proton energy deposition. The energy deposition of protons in matter exhibits the Bragg peak effect (Figure 5.19). Bragg peak is used to describe the energy decay curve of particles passing through obstacles. The protons will not release a large amount of energy immediately after entering the material. Only when the proton stops will it release most of its energy, forming a sharp energy peak — Bragg peak. The thickness we select can avoid the energy peak of protons and thus excessive heat deposition on the target material.

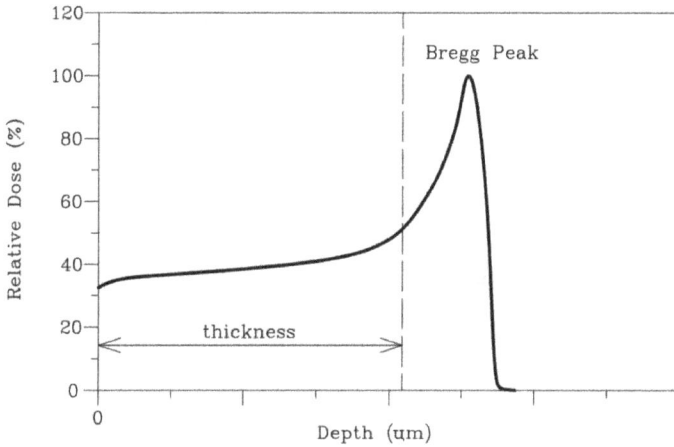

Figure 5.19   Bragg peak of proton and thickness of target material.

5.2.3.3.4 Heat Dissipation of Target

A key factor that affects the performance and lifetime of a target system is the heat dissipation. When a proton beam is incident on the target, the nuclear reaction with the target material results in a loss of energy. Almost all the energy of the proton will be converted into heat deposited in the target. In general, in order to meet the treatment requirements of BNCT, the power of the proton accelerator should reach tens of kilowatts. If a low-energy proton beam is used to bombard the lithium target, it needs to reach a high current intensity. If a beryllium target is bombarded, the proton beam intensity does not need to be too high, but it does require high energy. Thus in any case, the total heat load deposited in the target will be tens of kilowatts, equivalent to the power of the accelerator.

Due to the insufficient strength and rigidity of the target material, it needs to be placed on other supporting metals, such as copper, stainless steel, etc. Liquid channels can be arranged on the supporting metal to eliminate the thermal load of the target system by means of liquid cooling and heat conduction. The most commonly used heat transfer medium is water. The cooling efficiency can be improved by special cooling channel design or increasing the cooling water flow. Materials with high thermal conductivity must also be used as a part of the target system or its auxiliary parts.

At the same time, it is necessary to reduce the unit heat load of the proton beam loaded on the target surface, which can be achieved by enlarging the proton beam spot with magnets at the exit port of the accelerator. It is also possible to change the shape of the target from flat to conical or other shapes. Multiple targets can also be arranged on a ring-shaped rotating structure and successively irradiated by the proton beam. Essentially, these are all about reducing the heat load per unit area by increasing the contact area between the proton beam and the target material.

5.2.3.3.5 Blistering of Target

Protons stopped in the metal are converted to hydrogen gas by taking free electrons from the metal. When the concentration of hydrogen gas reaches a certain amount, the metal will be broken by the blistering. This makes the target fragile and short-lived, affecting the BNCT treatment process. This is an inevitable problem for neutron-generating targets using proton beams. Protons will eventually deposit somewhere to obtain free electrons and turn into hydrogen gas.

One solution is to use a higher-energy proton beam, such as 30 MeV or above. Protons are deposited in cooling water at the end of the target system, not in the target material, turn into hydrogen gas and are taken away by the water. When the proton beam energy is low, other methods should be considered. If protons are inevitably deposited in the target, metals with high hydrogen absorption, such as palladium and vanadium, can be arranged in the deposition position.

5.2.3.3.6 Activation of Target Material

In addition, charged particles incident on the target will cause activation. After protons bombard the lithium, the radioactive product ^{7}Be will be produced. Due to its long yield and half-life, this product is dangerous and requires special handling. Since the life cycle of the target is much shorter than that of the whole accelerator system, and there are inevitable activation problems, the target is usually made to be replaceable at any time. The methods to handle target activation problems include: remote control of target replacement by manipulator, and storage of abandoned target in lead tank; making a sealed target structure that cannot leak radioactive products to the outside, and replacing it for special storage and treatment after the target life expires; removal of lithium and the reaction products on the supporting metal with flowing water, and setting up of a wastewater tank for storage and treatment.

5.2.3.3.7 Comparison between Lithium and Beryllium Targets

This section introduces the characteristics of neutron-generating targets. Table 5.7 summarizes the advantages and disadvantages of lithium and beryllium targets.

5.2.3.4 *Beam Shaping Assemblies*

In the current accelerator-based neutron sources for BNCT, the protons are generally accelerated to about 2 MeV or even tens of MeV and

Table 5.7 Comparison between lithium and beryllium targets.

	Lithium Target	Beryllium Target
Advantages	Low energy requirement for proton accelerator and cost-saving.	High melting point, high thermal conductivity and low heat dissipation difficulty.
	The generated neutron energy spectrum is better and the moderating cost is saved.	Relatively easier to process and manufacture, longer service life.
Disadvantages	Low melting point, low thermal conductivity and difficult heat dissipation. May cause lithium evaporation and affect the generation of neutrons.	Relatively higher energy requirement for proton accelerator and higher cost.
	Produce radioactive products.	Toxic.
	Poor mechanical properties, active chemical properties, difficult to handle.	The neutron energy generated is higher, so the moderator is larger in size and higher in cost.

bombard the target materials such as lithium and beryllium. And then the maximum energy of the neutrons released by the target materials ranges from several hundreds of keV to tens of MeV. These neutrons are fast neutrons which are inapplicable for BNCT. Thus, the fast neutrons must be moderated and filtered to epithermal neutrons suitable for treatment. The neutron intensity is recommended as 1×10^9 (n/cm^{2}s) or higher, but that amount from the target material is not abundant for many current ABNSs. Therefore, a suitable moderator for the beam shaping assembly (BSA) that enables effective generation of epithermal neutrons should be designed specifically. The generated neutrons must be moderated to a suitable energy spectrum for BNCT after passing through the BSA.

The overall design of the BSA needs to use the Monte Carlo neutron transport[7] program to carry out multiple optimization calculations to determine the optimal solution, in order to meet the IAEA-recommended parameters range as the termination condition for the optimal design. This is a relatively strict index, and many current equipment and design schemes rarely fully meet the requirements of this index.

Like the neutron moderator mentioned in Section 5.1.6, the BSA system of the BNCT neutron irradiation system is based on the same principle. The difference from the reactor is the energy required for moderation and the quality of the exit neutron beam are different, but the most basic function is to reduce the energy of fast neutrons to epithermal neutrons.

The BSA also needs the ability to cut and filter low-energy neutrons (thermal neutrons) and γ rays contained in the epithermal neutron beam in addition to the reduction of high-energy neutrons (fast

---

[7] Neutron transport refers to the study of neutron-material interactions. Increasingly challenging problems in the nuclear industry require higher computational power and more accurate approximations. Two main branches of approach, deterministic method and stochastic method, are used in neutron transport calculations today. In particular, Monte Carlo simulation, as a stochastic method, has been widely used. The Monte Carlo methods approach the neutron transport problem by simulating the interactions of individual neutrons with high detail from their birth to the eventual absorption or leakage of the neutron.

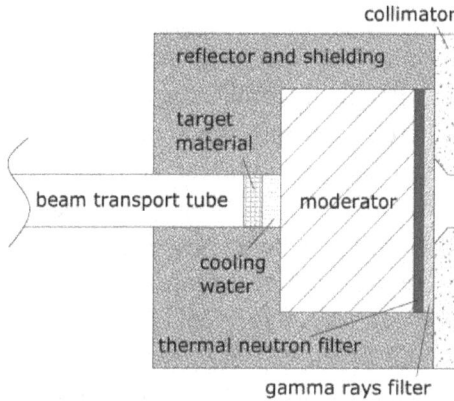

Figure 5.20 A schematic diagram of the BSA system. Reproduced with permission from http://www.jsnct.jp/pdf/bpa-bnct20200217_2.pdf.

neutrons). Furthermore, we have to also consider shielding all radiations leaking from the walls outside the beam aperture as much as possible.

Figure 5.20 shows a schematic diagram of the BSA system located behind the target. BSA is mainly composed of moderator, filter, reflector and collimator. Select the appropriate materials for each part according to its function, and then the size is optimized. At the same time, we try to meet the conditions of appropriate cost, simple design, easy manufacturing and installation, and convenient maintenance.

(1) *Moderator*

The role of the moderator is to moderate high-energy fast neutrons to lower-energy epithermal neutrons. Moderating materials should have small atomic mass number, low neutron absorption cross-section, high scattering cross-section for fast neutrons and low scattering cross-section for epithermal neutrons. At the same time, the moderator material should also have a low radiation capture cross-section and a low γ emissivity to avoid the harm of γ radiation damage to the patient. The moderation effect depends more on the material geometry. As the thickness increases, the flux ratio of epithermal neutrons to fast neutrons will increase, but the most important parameter, the epithermal neutron flux, will decrease. Therefore, an optimization of the thickness is required.

For materials with large atomic mass numbers, the energy lost by neutrons in collisions is too small to achieve the effect of moderation. Although materials with small atomic mass numbers are preferred, thermal neutrons will increase because the energy loss of neutrons in collisions with these materials is too great and too fast. Moreover, the radiation capture reaction cross-section of materials with small atomic mass numbers and neutrons is large, and γ rays are emitted. Therefore, unlike reactors, materials with too large and too small atomic mass numbers will not be considered for BNCT.

Moderate materials for BNCT are generally those of medium mass, such as Fluental (69% AiF_3 + 30% Al + 1% LiF, where LiF absorbs thermal neutrons and reduces the porosity of the material), Fe, Al, AlF_3, Al + AlF_3 (30% Al + 70% AlF_3), MgF_2, D_2O, graphite, *etc.* A high flux ratio of epithermal neutrons to fast neutrons can be obtained by optimizing the moderator thickness, *i.e.*, moderating more fast neutrons to epithermal neutrons.

Compared with Fluental, Al and AlF_3 have the disadvantage of low density. Thicker Al and AlF_3 are required to moderate the same neutrons. On the other hand, Al and AlF_3 have the advantage of being cheaper than Fluental. MgF_2 is also a good moderator for generating epithermal neutrons, with a relatively small mass number, a high scattering cross-section for fast neutrons, and less γ rays.

(2) *Filter*

If thermal neutrons are mixed into the irradiation beam, the dose on the skin surface will increase, so it is necessary to consider installing a thermal neutron shielding material behind the moderator. If γ rays are mixed into the irradiation beam, unnecessary dose will be increased, so it is necessary to consider installing γ ray shielding material behind the thermal neutron shielding material. The main function of the filter is to filter thermal neutron pollution and γ ray pollution, increase flux ratio of epithermal neutrons to thermal neutrons, flux ratio of epithermal neutrons to fast neutrons, and reduce γ dose. The filter layer material has a low epithermal neutron absorption cross-section, a high thermal neutron absorption cross-section, a high γ ray absorption cross-section, a low radiation capture cross-section, and a high scattering cross-section for fast neutrons. Generally, fast neutrons should not be captured but moderated to epithermal neutrons, otherwise epithermal neutron intensity in the irradiation beam would be too low. ^{3}He, ^{10}B, ^{6}Li, ^{14}N and Cl are better materials for filtering thermal neutrons. However, ^{3}He is a rare material, so it is not used. The more commonly employed is ^{6}LiF. Bi filters γ rays better than Pb, and the epithermal neutron absorption cross-section is smaller than that of Pb.

(3) *Reflector*

When protons bombard the target material, the generating neutrons are emitted from all directions around the target. Most of the high-energy neutrons travel forward, but some lower-energy neutrons scatter from the sides or back of the target. Therefore, in order to increase the neutron intensity of the irradiation beam, it is necessary to arrange reflectors on the side and back of the target to reflect the non-forward neutrons forward.

The function of the reflector is to reflect neutrons, avoid the leakage of neutrons, increase the flux of epithermal neutrons, and reduce the flux of fast neutrons; at the same time, guide the neutrons to the beam exit port. The material of the reflector desirably has a small neutron absorption cross-section and a large neutron scattering cross-section. Increasing the thickness of the reflector layer can increase the reflected neutron intensity, but it will increase the cost of shielding. Generally, the material of the reflector layer includes high atomic number materials such as Pb, Ni, Al, Bi, Al_2O_3 or graphite.

(4) *Collimator*

The function of the collimator is to make the neutron beam converge on the treated tumor area, that is, to focus and position the patient, so that the tumor can be better treated. The material should have a low absorption cross-section for epithermal neutrons. The collimator material is generally tungsten or lithiated polyethylene. Generally, a tapered channel structure is adopted.

It is also conceivable to mount the collimator behind the γ ray shielding material to reduce the dose outside the irradiation field.

However, since the intensity of neutrons may be reduced due to the installation of the collimator, more research is required.

The radiation leakage of BSA should be considered. One part is the out-of-field leakage in the beam exit surface, and the other part is the leakage in the rear surface. For the out-of-field neutron leakage, it is suggested to be less than 5% of the average beam intensity within the beam aperture at 10 cm away from the beam exit port, and less than 1% at a 30 cm distance. For the rear-end radiation leakage, it is recommended to be less than 10% of the main therapeutic neutron beam.

In addition, activation due to neutron incident on BSA should also be noted. Similar to the activation problem of the target, if the activation problem of BSA is serious, more shielding needs to be arranged, otherwise it may cause unnecessary doses to patients, physicians, and maintenance personnel.

The BSA shall minimize the composition of fast neutrons, thermal neutrons and γ rays, and ensure the directionality of epithermal neutrons. Its design and optimization is one of the core contents of the BNCT neutron source design.

The design of the BSA varies according to the proton energy and target material used, and the corresponding design is carried out according to the energy spectrum, flux, and angle of the emitted neutrons. For different systems, although each BSA has its unique design, the main components are similar, basically as described above. If geometric size of the BSA is too large and too many materials are used, it will lead to a high cost of construction. Similarly, if the activation problem is too serious, it will also cause great trouble for subsequent maintenance and handling of the system. However, at the current development stage of BNCT, the problems in this regard have not yet emerged, because the accelerator-based BNCT neutron generation systems have not been operated long enough.

5.2.3.5 *Accelerator-Based BNCT Facilities*

Several accelerator-based BNCT facilities are currently being designed and constructed for BNCT, some of which have been installed and tested at various centers in the world. Table 5.8 shows the current status and beam characteristics for accelerator BNCT facilities around the

Table 3.6 Current status and beam characteristics for accelerator BNCT facilities around the world.

Machine (Type)	Target	Beam Energy (MeV)	Beam Current (Actual/Design) (mA)	Facility (Location, Status)
C-BENS (Cyclotron)	^{9}Be(p, n) (thick 5.5 mm)	30	1(2)	Particle Radiation Oncology Research Center of Kyoto University (Kumatori, Japan, prototype/BNCT research)
NeuCure® (Cyclotron)				Southern Tohoku BNCT Research Center (Fukushima, Japan, patient treatment)
				Kansai BNCT Medical Center (Osaka Medical College, Osaka, Japan, patient treatment)
				BNCT Center in Hainan Boao Lecheng International Medical Tourism Pilot Zone (Hainan, China, under construction)
CICS-1 (RFQ Linac)	Solid ^{7}Li(p, n)	2.5	12(20)	National Cancer Center Hospital (Tokyo, Japan, phase I clinical trial)
				Edogawa Hospital BNCT Center (Tokyo, Japan, under construction)
iBNCT (RFQ+DTL Linac)	^{9}Be(p, n) (thick 0.5 mm)	8	2.1(10)	Ibaraki Neutron Medical Research Center (University of Tsukuba, Japan, experimental use)
A-BNCT (RFQ+DTL Linac)	^{9}Be(p, n)	10	8	Gachon University Gil Medical Center (Dawonsys, Incheon, Korea, preclinical trial)
NUANS (Dynamitron)	Solid ^{7}Li(p, n)	2.8	8(15)	Nagoya University (Nagoya, Japan, commissioning)

(Continued)

Table 5.8 (*Continued*)

Machine (Type)	Target	Beam Energy (MeV)	Beam Current (Actual/Design) (mA)	Facility (Location, Status)
nuBeam® (Electrostatic Single-ended DC)	Solid ^{7}Li(p, n)	2.6	30	Helsinki University Hospital (Helsinki, Finland, commissioning)
				Shonan Kamakura General Hospital (Kanagawa Prefecture, Japan, installing)
				High-Flux Accelerator-Driven Neutron Facility (Birmingham, UK, BNCT research/under construction)
				Institut Jules Bordet (University Hospital of Brussels, Brussels, Belgium, under construction)
NeMeSis (Electrostatic Single-ended DC)	Solid ^{7}Li(p, n)	2.6	30	Granada University Hospital (Granada, Spain, under construction)
VITA (Electrostatic Tandem)	Solid ^{7}Li(p, n)	2–2.3	10	Budker Institute of Nuclear Physics (Novosibirsk, Russia, prototype/BNCT research)
NeuPex™ (Electrostatic Tandem)	Solid ^{7}Li(p, n)	2.5	10	Xiamen Humanity Hospital (Xiamen, China, preclinical trial)
Alphabeam (Electrostatic Tandem)	Solid ^{7}Li(p, n)	2.5	10	Fondazione Centro Nazionale Adroterapia Oncologica (Pavia, Italy, under construction)

VITA (Electrostatic Tandem)	Solid ^{7}Li(p, n)	2.5	10	Blokhin National Medical Research Center of Oncology (Moscow, Russia, under construction)
ESQ (Electrostatic ESQ DC)	^{9}Be(d, n) (thin) ^{13}C(d, n) (thick)	1.45	7(30)	CNEA (Buenos Aires, Argentina, BNCT research/under construction)
KIRAMS AB-BNCT (Electrostatic)	—	—	—	Korea Institute of Radiological and Medical Sciences (Seoul, Korea, under construction)
D-BNCT01 (RFQ Linac)	^{9}Be(p, n)	3.5	10	Dongguan Neutron Science Center (Dongguan, China, BNCT research)
CYCIAE-14B (Cyclotron)	—	14	1	China Institute of Atomic Energy (Beijing, China, BNCT research/commissioning)
D-BNCT02 (RFQ Linac)	Solid ^{7}Li(p, n)	2.8	20	Dongguan People Hospital (Dongguan, China, under construction)
Mazu AB-BNCT (RFQ Linac)	—	—	—	Mazu Hospital (Fujian, China, commissioning)
Heron AB-BNCT (Cyclotron)	—	—	—	AB-BNCT at Hsinchu Biomedical Science Park (Heron Neutron Medical, Hsinchu, Taiwan, China, under construction)
Soreq (RFQ+DTL Linac)	Liquid ^{7}Li(p, n)	2.5	2(20)	Soreq Nuclear Research Center (Soreq, Israel, under development)
INFN-CNAO (RFQ Linac)	^{9}Be(p, n)	5	20–30	Legnaro National Laboratory, Italian Institute of Nuclear Physics (Pavia, Italy, under development)

world [52]. In addition to the facility and location, accelerator type, target material, and beam performance (including proton beam energy, target of beam current, and actual achieved value) are given. We discuss some of them in detail.

(1) *Southern Tohoku BNCT Research Center*
The system named "NeuCure®" consists of a cyclotron accelerator (HM-30, which was mentioned above), a beam transport system, a beam scanner system for heat reduction on the Be target, a target cooling system, a BSA, a collimator assembly, and a patient setup system. The main feature of the facility is that there were no serious technical challenges in the design. The cyclotron is a mature technology, and the target manufacturing process is simple. Since the incident proton beam on the target is stopped in the cooling water, the target has no blistering problem. On the other hand, high residual radiation level after long-term beam operation, which could be up to 100 msv/h or higher, needs to be addressed. Stray high-energy neutrons cause this. For the same reason, the BSA design was carried out carefully to keep the contamination of the epithermal neutrons by unwanted fast neutrons to within the allowed range.

Considering the results in terms of the neutron yield, thermal properties, and activation level, Be was selected as the target material. Table 5.9 shows the characteristics of Li, Be, Ta and W as target materials when irradiated by a 1 mA, 30 MeV proton beam [53].

In Table 5.9, neutron yield is high in the order of Be, Ta, Li and W. Due to the low melting point of Li, it is difficult to keep the Li target

Table 5.9   Target material property comparison of Li, Be, Ta and W with a 1 mA, 30 MeV proton beam.

Target	Melting Point (°C)	Boiling Point (°C)	Thermal Conductivity (W/m/K)	Neutron Yield (s/mA)	γ Ray Yield (s/mA)	γ Ray Yield per Neutron
Li	180	1,340	84.7	1.14E+14	9.80E+12	0.09
Be	1,278	2,970	201	1.90E+14	3.35E+12	0.02
Ta	3,017	5,458	57.5	1.27E+14	1.18E+14	0.93
W	3,422	5,555	174	9.65E+13	1.35E+14	1.40

stable under the irradiation of a proton beam of 30 kW power. Be has the highest neutron yield and thermal conductivity, smallest γ ray yield per neutron, and high melting point. In the system, beryllium target is cooled directly by pure compressed water, which flows through spiral graphite channels. Protons with a range of 5.8 mm in Be penetrate a 5.5 mm-thick Be target and inject in the compressed cooling water to prevent the target from blistering. According to the heat load test, for a heat input of 500 W/cm² leading to a temperature of less than 500°C, the irradiation area should be no less than 60 cm², under 30 kW operation. The irradiation area was expanded to 144 cm², which is sufficient for a heat input of 200 W/cm². Thus, a uniform 120 mm × 120 mm proton beam at the beryllium target is shaped by a controlling magnetic field of two scanning magnets. Another consideration for target is the activation, which was made as low as possible to avoid additional costs due to remotely operating equipment and heavy radiation shielding. Low activation is also important for hospital management in terms of maintenance, storage, and control of targets. Assuming 2 hours of irradiation per day with a proton current of 1 mA, target activation should be evaluated after one year of operation. Nuclei produced in W targets have higher activity and longer half-lives than Be and Ta targets. After one year of operation, the activation rate of the Ta target is 4 orders of magnitude higher than that of the Be target.

In order to treat a deep tumor, it is necessary to reduce the neutron energy to the range of epithermal energy. For this purpose, BSA is used in the system, which consists of moderator, reflector and thermal neutron filter. The moderator is used to reduce neutron energy from 28 MeV to low capture cross-section. Pb and Fe are the common moderator materials. Pb has a cross-section of about 1 barn for the (n,2n) reaction with the maximum neutron energy greater than 10 MeV. In addition, for incident neutron energies greater than 1 MeV, the inelastic scattering cross-section of Pb is approximately 1 barn. The (n,2n) reaction cross-section of Fe is smaller than Pb, but the inelastic scattering cross-section of Fe is larger than Pb at incident neutron energies of several MeV. Therefore, the Pb component was installed near the target area, and the Fe component was installed after the Pb component. The Pb component was placed as a reflector around the Be target assembly to reflect neutrons that are backscattered by the Be target. The target

Table 5.10 Beam property of CBNS (NeuCure®) under free-air condition compared with KUR epithermal mode.

	Epithermal Neutron Flux, Φ_{epi} (n/cm²/s)	Fast-Neutron Dose, D_f/Φ_{epi} (Gy·cm²/n)	γ Ray Dose, D_γ/Φ_{epi} (Gy·cm2/n)
KUR (epithermal)	7.30E+08	9.10E–13	2.40E–13
Accelerator	1.88E+09	5.84E–13	7.75E–14

assembly is removable for easy target replacement. Thermal neutron filter is used to obtained optimal neutron energy into the thermal energy range, which is made of Al and CaF_2 in the system. The combination of Al and F limits the neutron energy to around 27 keV. Although the commonly used materials are AlF_3 and FLUENT™ (composed of 69% AlF_3, 30% Al, and 1% ^6LiF, developed by the Finnish company VTT), it is difficult to make a compact BSA with these because the density of AlF_3 is difficult to increase, because it sublimates under atmospheric pressure at a temperature of 1,040 °C. Therefore, Al and CaF_2 are used instead of AlF_3.

The fast-neutron and γ ray dose contaminations per epithermal neutron for CBNS (NeuCure®) under the free-air condition and those for KUR are shown in Table 5.10. In this regard, the CBNS facility is superior to KUR.

Epithermal neutrons pass through the BSA and lead to a collimator assembly, which is placed behind a γ shield made of Pb. The collimator consists of natural LiF-loaded polyethylene blocks with a thickness of 1.5 cm. The collimator aperture can be adjusted to a radius of 25 cm and formed into any shape to fit the irradiation field. The patient can sit easily and insert the foot into the cone of the collimator.

To protect the patient from exposure to fast neutron radiation, the BSA (especially the front surface of the collimator) are surrounded by polyethylene blocks. These polyethylene blocks also serve as a shield around the irradiation room. To help the patient adopt a comfortable irradiation posture, the irradiation bed can be moved left and right, or up and down, or back and forth. The irradiation bed and the collimator assembly can also be moved backwards, and before starting the irradiation, the irradiation area can be confirmed by a view taken from the beam direction through the collimator aperture. This backward movement is also used to measure the neutron spectrum under free-air conditions in order to establish neutron sources for treatment planning.

In addition, an X-ray tube and imaging plate are installed in order to accurately set the patient in the position determined by the treatment planning system. The irradiation position is determined by comparing the bone image (reconstructed from the CT image) obtained through the treatment plan with the X-ray image of the imaging plate. By moving a pair of X-ray tubes and imaging plate to the side of the neutron beam, an image of the "beam's eye view" can be obtained. A laser marking machine is also installed; the irradiation position is determined by the markings on the skin.

In the Southern Tohoku BNCT Research Center (Figure 5.21), the treatment room has a unique design, differing from that of the prototype machine C-BENS, with two rooms of the same specifications, and the beam quality equivalency was confirmed in both rooms. Both treatment rooms feature horizontal beamlines to facilitate patient setup and reduce construction costs. A BNCT facility with multiple treatment rooms in a hospital has limited space. Remote Patient Carrying System requires a straight track between the preparation and treatment rooms, resulting in limited layout of these rooms. A patient was set up in the preparation room located in front of the treatment room and the method of transporting the patient to the treatment room remotely was used as a basic workflow. Adopting this approach eliminates the need for medical staff to work in the activated treatment room immediately after exposure, and ensures sufficient distance from the treatment room to reduce the cumulative exposure for medical staff. Finally, the beamline configuration was designed as an upside-down Y-shape with all these issues in mind, in which the accelerator and two treatment rooms are located on the top and bottom, respectively. Based on the patient flow, workflow, and setup of the preparation room, the optimal layout was determined to be a beam deflection angle of 55° [72].

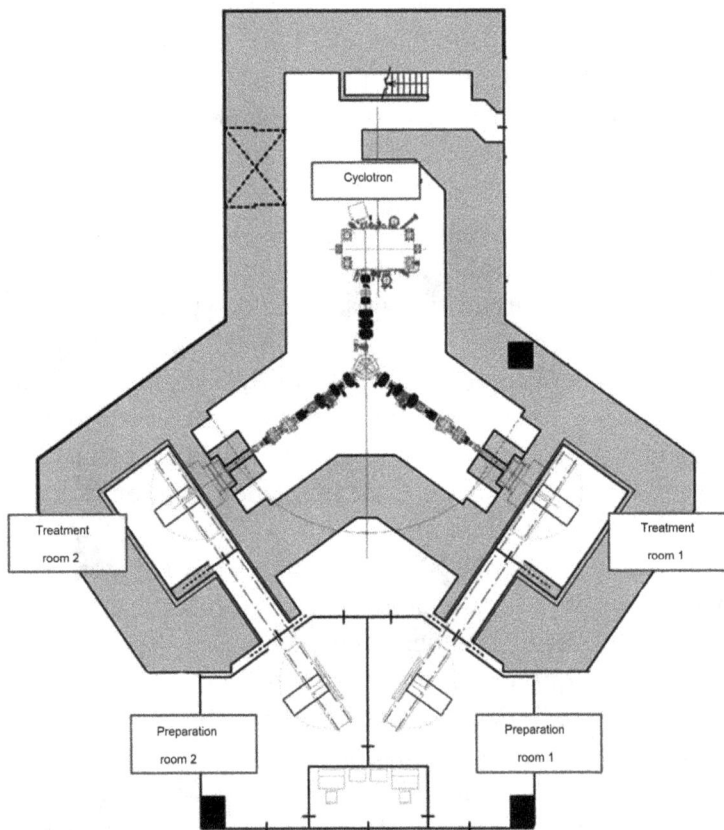

Figure 5.21 Schematic layout of the basement floor of the Southern Tohoku BNCT Research Center [72].

(2) *Helsinki University Hospital*

Helsinki University Hospital and NTI formed a joint project to install a compact ABNS in the campus area of the University Hospital of Helsinki (Figure 5.22). The facility was designed and constructed under the supervision of appropriate regulatory and international recommendations [1]. The facility is connected to other hospital buildings by a service tunnel and has two floors. The acceleration room, treatment room, control room and patient preparation room are located on the ground floor, and the supporting laboratory is located on the upper floor. Since the facility is located within the hospital campus, hospital resources and infrastructure are available for patient care [55].

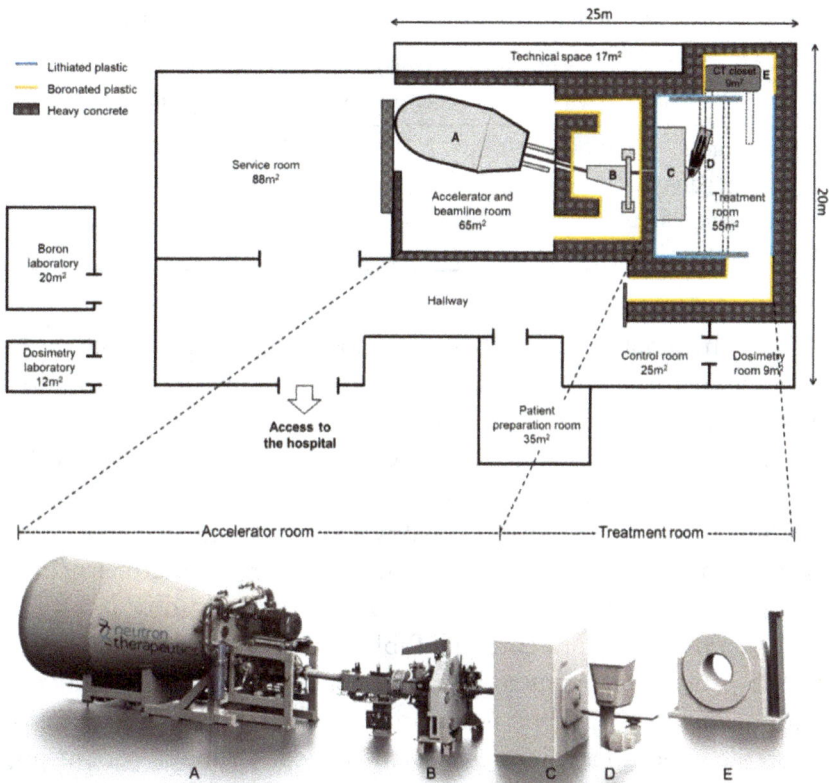

Figure 5.22 The general layout of the BNCT facility in Helsinki (upper). The accelerator, neutron source system and treatment room are located on the ground floor. Laboratories and offices are located upstairs and are only accessible to personnel. Neutron source system based on the nuBeam® compact accelerator (lower). From left to right: (A) proton accelerator, (B) proton beam optics, (C) beam shaping assembly, (D) robotic couch, and (E) rail-mounted CT [55].

The neutron source system, nuBeam® mentioned above, is an accelerator-based in-hospital neutron source to replace nuclear reactors. The system consists of a single-ended 2.6 MeV, 30 mA electrostatic proton accelerator, a beam transport system, an on-line proton beam monitoring system, a rotating solid Li target for neutron generation with reaction ^{7}Li(p,n)^{7}Be, a BSA, and an on-line neutron beam monitoring system. Circular beam delimiter sizes vary from 8 cm to 20 cm and are nominally 14 cm in diameter. The on-line neutron beam monitoring detectors are placed inside the BSA embedded in the beam

Table 5.11   Beam parameters of nuBeam® compared with FiR 1.

	Φ_{epi} (n/cm²/s)	D_f/Φ_{epi} (Gy·cm²/n)	D_γ/Φ_{epi} (Gy·cm²/n)	Φ_{th}/Φ_{epi}	J/Φ_{epi}
FiR 1 (measured)	1.1E+09	2.3E–13	5.0E–14	0.0673	0.77
nuBeam (MCNP6) 14 cm beam, 30 mA, 100% neutron yield	1.5E+09	1.9E–13	4.0E–14	0.012	0.73

delimiter material so that they can observe the epithermal beam. Depending on the neutron flux reported by the beam monitors, the treatment dose is controlled by automatically terminating the irradiation. This provides a more direct measurement of the delivered dose than relying on the calibrated proton current data.

The design of the neutron beam was similar to the neutron source beam based on the FiR 1 reactor, aiming at high epithermal neutron flux, as well as low fast neutron, thermal neutron and γ dose levels. The beam parameters are presented in Table 5.11.

The patient treatment room meets applicable standards in medical facilities, including patient monitoring and temperature, ventilation, and sterile conditions. Since the beam is fixed, a robotic patient positioning and image-guiding system, Exacure made by BEC GmbH (Reutlingen, Germany), was installed in the treatment room. In-room imaging is performed using a rail-mounted Siemens Healthineers Somatom Confidence RV CT scanner. The patient preparation room, located next to the treatment room, is used for physical examinations, boron infusion and blood sampling. A pneumatic transmission tube was installed for the rapid transfer of the blood samples to the boron laboratory.

For radiation safety, the accelerator room and treatment room are classified as controlled areas, the control room and patient preparation room as supervision areas, and those working in the facility are considered Class A radiation personnel.

(3) *National Cancer Center Hospital*
As a solution, CICS installed an accelerator-based neutron capture therapy facility at the NCC to generate neutrons from ^{7}Li(p,n)^{7}Be nuclear

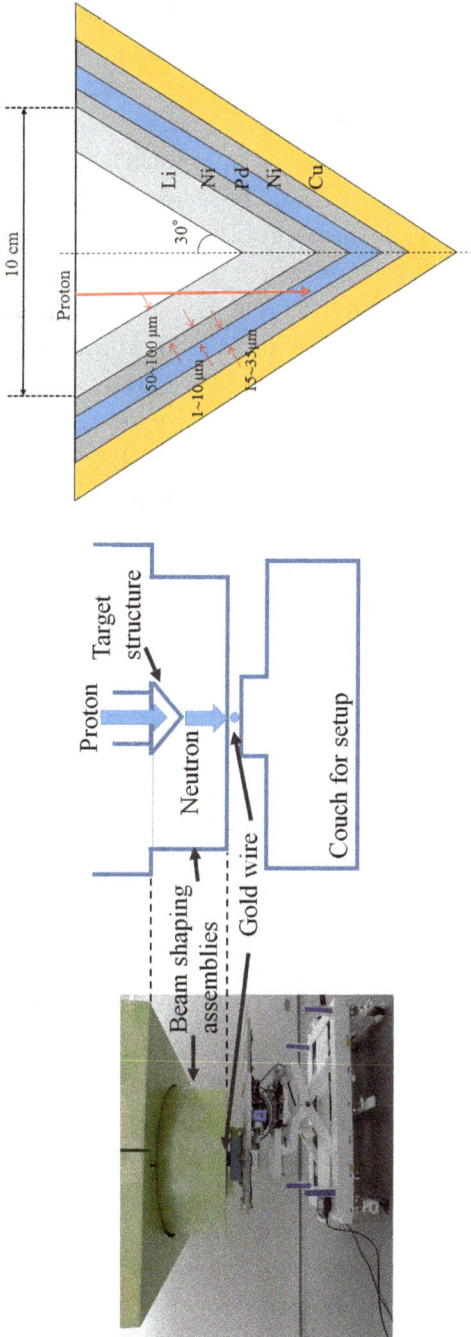

Figure 5.23 Schematic of the NCC facility configuration (left) and target system (right) [99].

reactions by using a 2.5 MeV proton beam on a solid Li target. A schematic of the system is shown in Figure 5.23 (left). To meet the neutron flux requirement for BNCT, a 20-mA high current proton beam is required. Therefore, the heat load at the Li target becomes 50 kW, causing blistering to be an issue. Furthermore, after long-term beam operation, it is necessary to avoid the accumulation of radioactive elements, such as ^{7}Be and tritium. CICS solved these problems by designing an automatic regeneration device for Li target. Three rotary port mechanisms are used to achieve automatic reforming Li layer. The first port is used for irradiation normally. The second port is used to strip off the Li layer with water, here taking advantage of the "problem" that Li reacts strongly with water. The residual is drained off and stored in a storage tank at hospital premises. The third port is used for generating a new Li layer by vapor deposition [100]. The target structure consists of a thin solid-state Li target, a first Ni layer, a Pd layer, a second Ni layer, and a copper support. Their thicknesses are 50.0, 3.0, 14.0, 7.0, and 10.0×10^2 μm, respectively. A schematic of the target structure is shown in Figure 5.23 (right).

5.3 Dosimetries in BNCT

5.3.1 Dose Composition and Evaluation

Among the doses generated by the neutron beam which is irradiated into the human body, the boron dose with therapeutic effect generated by the nuclear reaction between ^{10}B and thermal neutrons is the most dominant. Other doses generated by the nuclear reactions between the neutrons and hydrogen/nitrogen elements that make up biological tissues are inevitable, and are called background doses or non-boron doses. In addition, the primary γ rays mixed in the neutron beam and the secondary γ rays generated by the nuclear reaction between neutrons and biological tissues can also cause unnecessary doses to the human body. All of these doses need to be evaluated, to assess the damage and total dose delivered to each tissue and lesion by irradiation. Since the biological effects of each absorbed dose are different, the equivalent dose is estimated by multiplying each absorbed dose by the corresponding RBE factor. In addition, even in a region uniformly irradiated with neutron rays at the macroscopic level (medical image level), the doses generated in this region are completely different because of the different distribution of ^{10}B at the microscopic level (cellular level). Tumor killing effect depends on the uptake and distribution of ^{10}B in cancer cells. Therefore, according to the boron agent used and the type of tissue, different Compound Biological Effectiveness (CBE)[8] factors are selected to be multiplied by the boron dose to calculate the equivalent dose. Dose assessment of BNCT needs to be performed for each tumor and tissue separately.

(1) *Boron dose*

The effective dose of BNCT comes from the energy that the ^{10}B(n, α)^{7}Li nuclear reaction emits after ^{10}B atoms absorbs thermal neutrons, and the generated α and Li particles are deposited in the tissue. The dose largely depends on the distribution of ^{10}B in the organism, especially the ratio of the concentration of ^{10}B in the tumor to that in the blood, the absolute concentration in the tumor tissue, and the micro-distribution in the cells (even if the ^{10}B is captured by the tumor cell, it could be distributed unevenly between inside and outside the nucleus).

In practical clinical applications, the concentration of ^{10}B in tumor tissues is preferably several times that of normal tissue (up to 2.5

---

[8] The concept of RBE is valid only when the quantity of absorbed dose can be defined, i.e., when the averaging procedure implicit in the definition of absorbed dose is applicable. For the boron dose in BNCT, the concept of absorbed dose cannot be applied because of the inhomogeneous distribution of the boron compounds and the short range of the α and lithium particles. Therefore, the RBE cannot be defined and the influence of an inhomogeneous distribution of the boron atoms cannot be determined. Only the product of these two components, RBE and boron distribution, can be assessed for a given tissue and experimental conditions.

The CBE factor is a conversion factor that converts the physical dose from the boron neutron capture reaction ^{10}B(n, α)^{7}Li to the biological X-ray equivalent dose. All CBE factors currently used in biological tissues are derived from animal experiments and clinical trials. It is important to understand the CBE factor because it is directly related to the BNCT principle. Different compounds have different CBEs, and a CBE factor needs to be determined for each boron drug used in BNCT.

or more), and the content of ^{10}B in tumor cells should reach about $20 \sim 35$ µg ^{10}B/g tumor. To achieve a good therapeutic effect at this concentration, a thermal neutron flux of 1×10^{12} (n/cm^2)[9] is required.

Boron drugs might accumulate in normal tissues of the skin and mucous membranes, but this is undesired. Therefore, in the evaluation of the boron dose, the doses of tumor cells and each normal tissue (skin, brain, mucous membranes, *etc.*) must be evaluated separately.

(2) Non-boron dose

The non-boron dose has nothing to do with the boron in normal cells or tumor cells, but is incidentally generated by neutron radiation with the human tissue.

a) Hydrogen dose (fast neutron dose), D_f
The energy deposited in the local tissue by the recoil protons generated by the ^{1}H(n, n')p reaction between epithermal and fast neutrons colliding with hydrogen atoms in the tissue reaches a maximum in the skin and superficial tissue, and then decline exponentially. Decreased D_f reduces skin damage.

b) Nitrogen dose (thermal neutron dose), D_N
The energy deposited in the local tissue by the 600 keV protons and recoil nuclear ^{14}C particles generated by the capture reaction ^{14}N(n, p)^{14}C between thermal neutrons and nitrogen atoms in the tissue.

c) γ dose, D_γ
The primary γ ray dose generated by the neutron irradiation system and the 2.2 MeV secondary γ ray dose generated by the ^{1}H(n, γ)^{2}H reaction between thermal neutrons and hydrogen atoms in the tissue.

---

[9] Assuming that the concentration of ^{10}B in tumor cells is 25 µg ^{10}B/g tumor, the concentration in tumor/normal ratio is 3.5, so the CBE factor of the tumor is recommended to be 3.8. The thermal neutron flux irradiating the tumor is 1×10^{12} n/cm^2, thus the equivalent X-ray dose generated by the nuclear reaction between ^{10}B and thermal neutrons will be about 25 Gy-eq.

(3) *Calculation of absorbed dose*
The absorbed dose, D_n, due to the reaction between the neutron and each element is calculated according to Eq. (5.2).

$$D_n = \iint K_n(E)\varphi(E,t)dEdt \qquad (5.2)$$

where $K_n(E)$ is the neutron Kerma factor and $\varphi(E, t)$ is the neutron beam flux. The Kerma factor is the sum of the initial kinetic energies of the secondary charged particles released within the cell by indirectly ionized particles,[10] such as neutrons. The process of dose generation by indirect ionized particles in matter can be divided into two steps: (1) indirect ionized particles interact with matter to generate charged particles and secondary indirect ionized particles; (2) the generated charged particles are ionized and excited to generate dose in the tissue. The Kerma factor is the result of the first step and absorbed dose is the result of the second step. However, indirect ionization of particles in matter to release energy to charged particles and then charged particles to release energy to matter do not necessarily occur at the same location. The Kerma factor varies according to the neutron energy. Also, for each element (hydrogen, nitrogen, boron), the Kerma factor is different. Therefore, when calculating the absorbed dose using Eq. (5.2), the dose in each evaluation point needs to be multiplied by the Kerma factor corresponding to each neutron energy and nuclear reaction.

In addition, the neutron beams used in BNCT are neutrons with a certain energy range. After being irradiated into the patient's body, the neutron energy spectrum of different positions differs. For example, when an epithermal neutron beam is used, the skin surface is directly

---

[10] Photons and neutrons are "indirectly ionizing" (as compared to α and β particles that are "directly ionizing") forms of radiation. So, γ rays and neutrons are indirectly ionized particles. In addition, with regard to boron dose, the distribution of ^{10}B in tumor cells and normal tissues differs, and the concentration changes over time. The boron dose received per 1 ppm should be obtained by using the Kerma factor per 1 ppm boron concentration, and then multiplied by the total boron concentration of the target tissue to obtain the boron dose.

irradiated, and the neutron energy spectrum here is basically the same as the beams coming out of the treatment port. For the neutrons entering the living body and reacting with the biological tissues, they slow down, making the proportion of lower-energy neutrons (thermal neutrons) increase, and the neutron flux gradually decreases. So, the neutron flux used in Eq. (5.2) must be the neutron flux corresponding to the neutron energy at each point to be evaluated.

In general, the calculation of neutron absorbed dose is too complicated and cumbersome. In the dose assessment of BNCT, the absorbed dose of each element is usually estimated by using the method of Monte Carlo Neutron Transport.

(4) Calculation of equivalent dose
In order to estimate the total dose applied to a patient through neutron irradiation, it is necessary to multiply the absorbed dose value of each dose by the corresponding RBE or CBE factor, and add them to obtain the Equivalent Dose (hereinafter referred to as ED). Use "Gy-Eq" as the unit of equivalent dose. The efficacy of BNCT can be assessed by comparing equivalent dose with other radiation treatments such as X-ray therapy. The formula for calculating the equivalent dose is shown in Eq. (5.3).

$$ED(G_\gamma-Eq) = C_B \times D_{B,1PPm} \times CBE_B + D_N \times RBE_N + D_f \times RBE_f$$
$$+ D_\gamma \times RBE_\gamma \tag{5.3}$$

where C_B is the ^{10}B concentration (ppm), and CBE_B, RBE_N, RBE_f, and RBE_γ correspond to the CBE and RBE factors of the absorbed doses, respectively. In addition, tumor cells and normal tissues have different CBE factors, which further change with different boron agents. Typical RBE factors for non-boron doses are recorded in Table 5.12.

The CBE factor is a coefficient for converting the boron dose to the biological X-ray dose, as shown in Eq. (5.3). The currently used CBE factor of normal tissues are obtained through cell and animal experiments. When calculating the CBE factor of normal tissue, the C_B corresponding to Eq. (5.3) uses the boron concentration in the blood. At present, there is no method to measure the boron concentration in

Table 5.12   Typical RBE factors for non-boron doses.

Absorbed Dose	RBE Factor
Hydrogen dose (fast neutron dose), D_f	2.0–3.2
Nitrogen dose (thermal neutron dose), D_N	2.5–3.2
γ dose, D_γ	1.0

Table 5.13   CBE factors used in BNCT based on Japanese reactors.

		Brain	Skin	Oral Mucosa	Lung
Boron dose, D_B	BSH	0.37	0.8	0.3	—
	BPA	1.35	2.5	4.3	2.3

tumor and normal tissues in real time during irradiation. The only sample that can measure boron concentration in patients is blood. Therefore, in order to use Eq. (5.3) for dose evaluation clinically, it is recommended to use the boron concentration in blood collected before irradiation. The boron concentration in blood is measured using devices like Inductively Coupled Plasma (ICP) emission spectrometer. Table 5.13 shows the CBE factors used when conducting BNCT using Japanese reactors.

The dose limit of normal tissue is 12.5 Gy, and the dose of tumors should be increased as much as possible within this limit range during irradiation. At the same time, skin dose exceeding 11 Gy should be avoided, and should be minimized as much as possible.

5.3.2 Neutron Beam Performance Evaluation

Although the configuration of the proton accelerator, neutron generating target, BSA and other parts used in different accelerator-based BNCT devices are not the same, at the treatment beam port the characteristic parameters of the final therapeutic epithermal neutron beams, such as neutron beam intensity distribution, energy spectrum distribution, angle distribution, and treatment beam quality parameters, can be unified. Neutron sources with similar characteristic parameters can

191

generate equivalent macroscopic distributions of secondary radiation fields in patients' bodies.

IAEA-TECDOC-1223 [2] is recommended as an index for BNCT neutron beam performance evaluation. The IAEA-TECDOC-1223 publication in 2001 by the IAEA gave the recommended range of parameters for the reactor neutron source for BNCT, which is a reference index for the design and development of BNCT neutron sources internationally. The detailed description of the parameters in Table 5.2 is as follows.

(1) *Epithermal neutron fluence rate* (Φ_{epi}): indicates the average density of epithermal neutrons that can reach the tumor site per second. This value determines the length of irradiation time required to achieve the prescribed dose. The larger the value, the shorter the time necessary for the patient to receive irradiation. When the value is greater than the IAEA recommended value, the irradiation time should be controlled to within one hour. For animal experiments, because the tumor is located in superficial tissues and the tumor volume is small, epithermal neutron flux greater than 10^8 can be permitted to meet the experimental requirements.

(2) *The ratio of neutron flux to neutron flux* (J/Φ) represents the directionality of the beam. The larger the ratio, the better the forward directivity of the neutron beam. A high forward neutron beam can reduce the dose to surrounding tissue caused by neutron emission and improve the treatment depth.

(3) *Fast neutron dose to epithermal neutron flux ratio* (D_f/Φ_{epi}), *thermal neutron to epithermal neutron flux ratio* (Φ_{th}/Φ_{epi}), γ *ray dose to epithermal neutron flux ratio* (D_γ/Φ_{epi}), *etc.*, belong to the "quality parameter" of the neutron source, which is used to guide the optimal design of the BSA. However, the quality parameters of neutron beams have certain differences between different neutron sources. Quality parameters of neutron sources are "microscopic parameters", which do not directly demonstrate the safety of BNCT. In other words, there is no clear quantitative relationship between effect in BNCT and the severity of complications. Generally, the macroscopic performance of the neutron source

quality is evaluated by the depth-dose distribution of the neutron beam in the phantom.[11]

However, when the IAEA-TECDOC-1223 recommendation index was determined for neutron beam performance evaluation, the main neutron source for BNCT was the reactor. Using previous indicators to guide the current design of accelerator-based neutron sources may not be very suitable. Some of the indicators are relatively hard to achieve, and there are few systems that are fully satisfied. Therefore, IAEA called for a meeting to assess the current status of the BNCT technique with emphasis on usage of compact accelerator-based intense neutron sources. The event also aimed to contribute to the update of IAEA-TECDOC-1223 in 2020 [66].

The neutron beam used by BNCT has a continuous energy spectrum distribution, and there are γ rays mixed in, so it is difficult to uniquely determine the beam performance. Therefore, in order to evaluate the performance of the neutron beam, it is necessary to perform dose evaluation through simulation of the phantom irradiation. Phantom parameters are used to study the therapeutic effect of the neutron beam in a patient, and to determine the therapeutic limit. It is said that a new revision of IAEA-TECDOC is being prepared, with dose assessment of the phantom being considered as one of the main criteria.

The parameters in the phantom are generally:

(1) *Advanced Depth* (AD): The depth at which the total dose received by the tumor is equal to the maximum allowable dose of normal

---

[11] Phantom materials include water, PMMA and brain tissue equivalent liquid (Liquid B). Liquid B has good consistency with the International Commission on Radiation Units and Measurements (ICRU) brain components. Water as a phantom medium shares similarity with the brain tissue in attenuating and scattering of epithermal neutrons. PMMA and water are commonly used as phantom materials in photon and BNCT dosimetry. The hydrogen concentration of PMMA is 14% lower than that of water or Liquid B, so the γ dose is consequently lower. However, the solid composition is appreciated in measuring practice. A phantom geometry is chosen to present a simple shape for establishing the dose calculations, but also as an approximate resemblance to the shape and size of the real patient and radiobiological object.

tissue. At the position after this depth, the tumor dose is less than the maximum allowable dose of normal tissue, losing the advantage of BNCT treatment. AD represents the penetrating ability of the neutron beam; the larger the AD, the deeper the tumor that can be treated. Its unit is cm.

(2) *Advantage Ratio* (AR): The ratio of the average dose received by tumor to normal tissue at a given depth (generally from the surface to AD). The average dose can be obtained by the integral of the depth-dose curve. The larger the AR, the better the therapeutic benefit of the neutron beam. Generally, AR $\geq$ 4 is required.

(3) *Therapeutic Depth* (TD): The depth at which the tumor dose drops to twice the maximum dose of normal tissue.

(4) *Advanced Depth Dose Rate* (ADDR): the tumor dose rate in AD, also equal to the maximum dose rate of normal tissue. Dose rate equals dose divided by treatment time. This parameter affects the length of treatment time. The larger the ADDR, the shorter the irradiation time needed to achieve the normal tissue tolerance dose.

(5) *Treatment Time*: The maximum allowable dose for normal tissue is 12.5 Gy, from which the treatment time can be obtained, preferably less than 1 hour in general.

As shown in Figure 5.24, AD is one of the most commonly used evaluation indicators. For tumor tissues with a depth less than AD, the dose received is greater than the maximum allowable dose of normal tissues. The greater the AD, the greater the ratio between the tumor dose and the normal tissue dose at the same depth (*i.e.*, the therapeutic gain). In the same way, the larger the AD, the deeper the tumor can be treated under the condition of a certain maximum dose of normal tissues.

BNCT and conventional radiotherapy have the following obvious differences:

(1) *Prescribed dose*: Conventional radiotherapy generally uses the target dose of the tumor as the prescription; however, currently BNCT generally uses the "skin tolerable dose" or "normal tissue tolerable dose" as the radiotherapy prescription, that is, the maximum

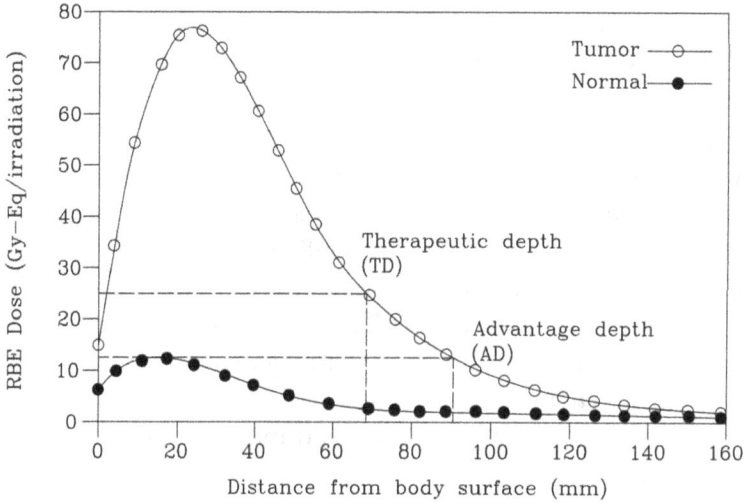

Figure 5.24 Typical depth-dose curve in BNCT [1].

allowable dose of the skin or normal tissue determines the irradiation plan.

(2) *Dose calculation*: The dose calculation of BNCT must use the Monte Carlo particle transport program to carry out detailed "mixed radiation field" simulation calculation, and to count the doses contributed by various nuclear reactions induced by neutrons, γ rays, and recoil protons. At the same time, the biological effects of each dose component must be considered.

(3) *Boron drug infusion*: The dose received by patients in BNCT is directly related to the microscopic distribution of boron drug in the target tissue, and the distribution of boron drug is closely related to the boron drug infusion scheme and drug metabolism.

5.3.3 *Neutron Detection*

As long as the energy and current intensity of the proton beam incident on the target, the state and structure of the target, and the material and structure of the BSA do not change, the neutron beam quality will basically not change. Since the dose of the nuclear reaction between [10]B and thermal neutrons dominates the therapeutically effective dose of BNCT, it is most important to determine the thermal neutron distribution in the phantom in confirming beam performance.

Because neutrons are electrically neutral particles, they are mainly subject to strong nuclear forces but not electric forces. Therefore, neutrons do not ionize directly, and they usually have to be converted into charged particles to be detected. Generally speaking, each type of neutron detector must be equipped with a converter (to convert neutron radiation to ordinary detectable radiation) and one of the conventional radiation detectors (scintillation detector, gaseous detector, semiconductor detector, *etc.*)

There are two basic types of neutron-matter interactions for neutron converters:

(1) *Elastic scattering*

Free neutrons can be scattered by the nucleus and transfer part of their kinetic energy to the nucleus. If the neutron has enough energy to scatter off nuclei, the recoil nucleus will ionize the material surrounding the converter. Only hydrogen and helium nuclei are light enough for practical application. The conventional detector can collect charges produced in this way to generate a detected signal. Neutrons can transfer more energy to light nuclei. This method is appropriate for detecting fast neutrons (fast neutrons have no high absorption cross-section), and can do so without moderators.

(2) *Neutron absorption*

This is a common method that allows the detection of neutrons throughout the energy spectrum. This method is based on various absorption reactions (radiative capture, nuclear fission, *etc.*). Neutrons are absorbed by the target material (converter) and emit secondary particles, such as protons, α particles, β particles, photons (γ rays) or fission fragments. Some are threshold reactions (requiring minimum energy of neutrons), but most reactions occur at epithermal and thermal energies. That means the moderation of fast neutrons is required, leading to poor energy information of the neutrons. The most common nuclei for the neutron converter material are:

- ^{10}B (n, α). Where the neutron capture cross-section for thermal neutrons is σ = 3,820 barns, and natural boron has an abundance of ^{10}B 19.8%.
- ^{3}He (n, p). Where the neutron capture cross-section for thermal neutrons is σ = 5,350 barns, and natural helium has an abundance of ^{3}He 0.014%.
- ^{6}Li (n, α). Where the neutron capture cross-section for thermal neutrons is σ = 925 barns, and natural lithium has an abundance of ^{6}Li 7.4%.
- ^{113}Cd (n, γ). Where the neutron capture cross-section for thermal neutrons is σ = 20,820 barns, and natural cadmium has an abundance of ^{113}Cd 12.2%.
- ^{235}U (n, fission). Where the fission cross-section for thermal neutrons is σ = 585 barns, and natural uranium has an abundance of ^{235}U 0.711%. Uranium as a converter produces fission fragments which are heavy charged particles. This has a significant advantage. The heavy charged particles (fission fragments) create a high output signal because the fragments deposit a large amount of energy in a detector-sensitive volume. This allows easy discrimination from the background radiation (e.g., γ radiation). This important feature can be used, for example, in a nuclear reactor power measurement, where a significant γ background accompanies the neutron field.

BNCT beams are complex mixed radiation fields, because of broad neutron energy range, presence of γ contamination and necessity of precise determination of several dose components.

In order to ensure the efficacy of the treatment and the safety of the patient, the characteristics of the radiation beam used must be determined before the treatment. The flux of the neutron and the dose accompanying the γ rays must be measured, as well as the absorbed dose in the phantom, which will help to develop an appropriate therapy plan. During the treatment, thermal and epithermal neutrons decay rapidly in the tissue, and the relative contributions of the four dose components vary significantly. The absorbed dose of the patient must be measured in real time to ensure the therapeutic effect. At present, two methods, cumulative dose measurement and real-time monitoring, are mainly used for dose measurement of BNCT.

The advantage of the cumulative dose measurement technique is the ability to accurately measure neutron and γ doses. The conventional measurement method is the gold foils/wires activation method, which measures the dose received by the patient. For example, when a gold wire is placed into a patient's body to a certain depth, thermal neutrons and gold undergo a nuclear reaction to produce radionuclides during the BNCT irradiation process. After a certain period of irradiation, the gold wire is taken out, and the activation reaction is measured. Then the boron concentration or neutron flux at the tissue where the gold wire was located can be reversed. In addition, thermoluminescent detectors are extensively used in BNCT due to their wide range, small size, reusability and high sensitivity.

(1) *Gold Foils/Wires Activation Method*
Use a material whose reaction cross-section has been accurately measured, put it into a certain point in the neutron field for measurement, irradiate it for a period of time, and take it out to measure the β or γ reflectivity it emits. The peak activity of the radionuclide formed in this material can be calculated according to the decay outline, thereby obtaining the neutron flux density.

But there is a disadvantage: it cannot continuously indicate the change of flux density over time. Because radionuclide formation is a cumulative process, and measurement and irradiation are separated in time, it is only suitable for measuring stable neutron flux densities.

Naturally occurring gold consists 100% of the isotope ^{197}Au. Gold is commonly used for neutron flux measurement since it has an appreciable thermal neutron absorption cross-section. The measurement technique is based on the neutron activation of gold foils/wires: ^{197}Au + n $\rightarrow$ ^{198}Au $\rightarrow$ ^{198}Hg + e$^-$ + γ. After capture of a neutron, ^{197}Au becomes ^{198}Au and emits a 411.8 keV γ ray. The β decay half-life of ^{198}Au is 2.6947 days. The initial gold activity can be calculated from the measured absolute γ intensity. And the neutron flux irradiated on gold foils/wires satisfies a certain formulaic relationship with the initial gold activity.

Activation of a gold foil/wire by a neutron spectrum is due to the total neutron quantity of both thermal and epithermal neutrons. It is possible to measure separately thermal and epithermal neutron fluxes by exposing one foil/wire to the neutron flux and exposing the same or another different foil/wire covered with cadmium (Cd), which will effectively block out the neutrons below the cadmium cut-off energy (0.4 eV). Therefore, the Cd-covered gold foil/wire will primarily be activated by epithermal neutrons.

Gold foils/wires can be placed at some specific positions in the phantom or the experimental subjects during the BNCT experiment. By measuring the γ rays from the gold foils/wires after the experiment with a high-purity germanium detector (HPGe detectors are the efficient solution for precise γ and X-ray spectroscopy), the neutron fluxes at those positions where the gold foils/wires used to be placed can be determined.

When using the activation method, it is necessary to understand that the measurement error is about 5%. The reasons include the radiation energy error of the standard radiation source when deriving the detection efficiency of the detector, the setting position error of the gold foils/wires, the measurement error of the balance used to measure the weight of the gold foils/wires, *etc.*

(2) *Neutron Thermoluminescent Dosimeter*
A thermoluminescent dosimeter, abbreviated as TLD, is a passive radiation dosimeter that measures ionizing radiation exposure *via* the intensity of visible light. The phenomenon of thermoluminescence was discovered in 1895 and TLDs were invented in 1954 by Professor Farrington Daniels of the University of Wisconsin-Madison, USA.

The following basic overview explains how the neutron TLD works:

a) Lithium fluoride (LiF) is a sensitive material used for γ and neutron radiation response.

b) Small crystals of LiF are the most common TLD chip material since they have the same absorption properties as soft tissue.

c) In the crystal of LiF, there are impurities (*e.g.*, manganese or magnesium), which produce trap states for trapping electrons in the band gap and holding them there. When the crystal is

199

exposed to the radiation, electrons are excited by ionization and will be captured in the trap states. With the absence of external excitation, the energetic electrons can stay there for a long time. This is equivalent to the crystal storing a part of the radiant energy received.

d) When the crystal is warmed, the trapped electrons are released and light is emitted. The amount of light is related to the dose of radiation received by the crystal. In order to obtain the dose received, the crystal must be heated in the TLD reader. The trapped electrons return to the ground state and emit photons of visible light. The amount of light emitted is called the glow curve.

e) The glow curve is analyzed to determine the dose. After reading all the curves we need, the TLD is annealed at a high temperature. This process essentially zeroes the thermoluminescent material by releasing all trapped electrons. The TLD is then ready for reuse.

f) Lithium has two stable isotopes, lithium-6 (7.4 %) and lithium-7 (92.6 %). ^{6}Li is the isotope sensitive to neutrons. The cross-section of ^{6}Li(n, α)^{3}H reaction for thermal neutrons is large, while that of ^{7}Li(n, γ)^{8}Li reaction for thermal neutrons is only $\sigma = 0.037$ barns. Therefore, the response of TLD-700 to thermal neutrons can be ignored.

g) The chip of TLD-600 is made of 95.6% ^{6}LiF and adds Mg and Ti as impurities. The chip of TLD-700 is made of 99.9% ^{7}LiF and adds Mg and Ti as impurities.

So, in the mixed radiation fields of BNCT, simultaneous use of TLD-700 measuring the γ ray dose and TLD-600 measuring the sum of γ ray dose and thermal neutron dose can enable calculation of the thermal neutron dose by subtracting them from each other.

Neither the gold foils/wires activation nor TLD detection are real-time dose monitoring methods, but rather are accumulated dose measurements.

(3) *Dual Ionization Chambers*
The ionization chamber is the simplest type of gas-filled radiation detector, which is widely used for the detection and measurement of certain types of ionizing radiation (Figure 5.25). An ionization

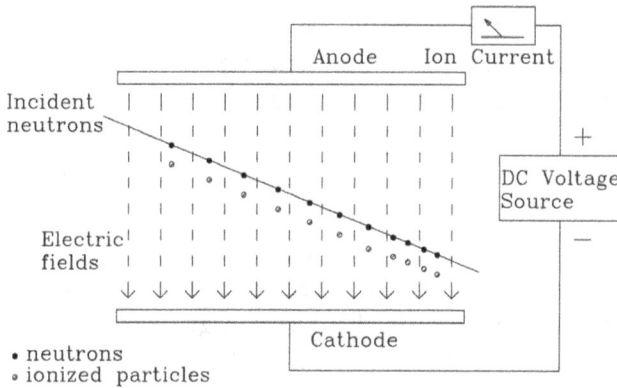

Figure 5.25 Visualization of an ion chamber operation. Reproduced with permission from https://instrumentationtools.com/ionization-chamber-principle/.

chamber measures the charge according to the number of ion pairs generated in the gas caused by incident radiation. It consists of a gas-filled chamber with two electrodes known as anode and cathode. A voltage potential is applied between the electrodes to generate an electric field in the gas. When gas atoms or molecules between the electrodes are ionized by incident ionizing radiation, ion pairs will be generated, and the resultant positive ions and dissociated electrons will move to the electrodes of the opposite polarity under the influence of the electric field. This produces an ionization current which is measured by an electrometer circuit. Each ion pair produced deposits or removes a small electric charge to or from an electrode, such that the accumulated charge is proportional to the number of ion pairs generated and therefore to the radiation dose. This continuously generated charge will produce an ionization current, which is a measure of the total ionization dose entering the chamber.

Because neutrons are electrically neutral particles, they will not be directly ionizing, and usually have to be converted into charged particles to be detected. One method for detecting neutrons using an ionization chamber is to coat with a thin layer of boron in the inner surface of the ionization chamber. When it is radiated by neutrons, $^{10}B(n, \alpha)^7Li$ reactions occur, accompanied by 0.48 MeV γ emission. The α particle causes ionization within the chamber, and ejected electrons will cause further secondary ionizations.

Another method is to use the gas boron trifluoride (BF_3) instead of air in the chamber. The incoming neutrons produce α particles when reacting with the boron atoms in the detector gas.

Based on ionization chamber technology, the photon beam profile in air and phantom can be measured, and the neutron and photon absorbed dose can also be measured. Many BNCT facilities worldwide have adopted the dual ionization chambers technology.

The technical concept of dual ionization chambers was first proposed by Attix, who used this technology to measure the neutron and γ doses of the mixed radiation field. MIT in the U.S., Petten in the Netherlands, and Finland have all used this technique to measure the mixed radiation field of BNCT. Usually, one of the ionization chambers is a tissue equivalent ionization chamber, whose response to γ and neutron is roughly the same; the other is a carbon graphite chamber that has a much larger response to γ than neutron. The wall of the tissue equivalent ionization chamber is made of tissue equivalent material, and the chamber is filled with tissue equivalent gas (64.4% CH_4, 32.5% CO_2, 3.1% N_2). The wall of the graphite ionization chamber is made of graphite, and the chamber is filled with carbon dioxide gas. The principle is to use two ionization chambers that have different responses to γ and neutron, and place them in a mixed radiation field for irradiation. After the current value of the dual ionization chamber is obtained, the doses of γ and neutron can be calculated according to Eqs. (5.4) and (5.5):

$$Q_{te} = A_{te}D_\gamma + B_{te}D_n$$
$$Q_{cg} = A_{cg}D\gamma + B_{cg}D_n$$

(5.4)

Where Q_{te} is the signal (current) collecting in the tissue equivalent ionization chamber;

Q_{cg} is the signal (current) collecting in the carbon graphite ionization chamber;

A_{te}, B_{te} are the responses to photons and neutrons, respectively, at the measurement point in the tissue equivalent ionization chamber;

A_{cg}, B_{cg} are the responses to photons and neutrons, respectively, at the measurement point in the carbon graphite ionization chamber; and

D_γ, D_n are the dose rate of photons and neutrons, respectively, at the measurement point. So:

$$D_\gamma = \frac{B_{te}Q_{cg} - B_{cg}Q_{te}}{B_{te}A_{cg} - B_{cg}A_{te}}$$

$$D_n = \frac{A_{te}Q_{cg} - A_{cg}Q_{te}}{A_{te}B_{cg} - A_{cg}B_{te}}$$

(5.5)

5.3.4 Treatment Planning

In the early 2000s, in the BNCT treatments using thermal neutrons with craniotomy, irradiation conditions were determined based on an evaluation of the actual measured dose. But for BNCT based on epithermal neutron beams, the treatment planning process is basically the same as that of the conventional X-ray therapy and particle beam therapy. A dedicated treatment planning system (TPS) is required in BNCT to produce dose plans/prescription dose and/or neutron flux to the patient, where all the mixed-field characteristics of the epithermal beam have been taken into account. Since neutrons are involved, the best method for calculating dose and flux in complex patient geometries is based on Monte Carlo. The dose evaluation process of the BNCT TPS is shown in Figure 5.26. A list of the available BNCT TPSs is presented in Table 5.14.

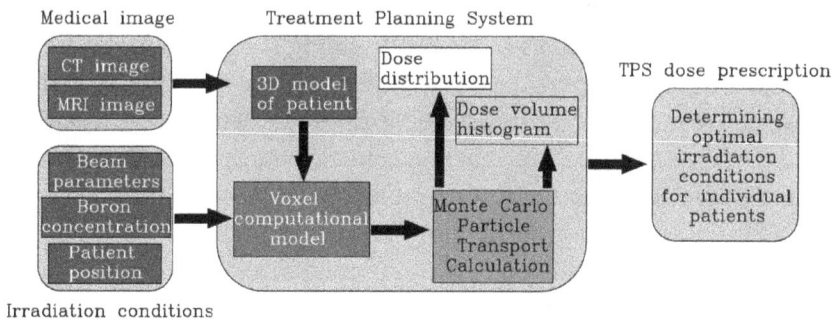

Figure 5.26   The dose evaluation flow of the BNCT treatment planning system.

Table 5.14   The BNCT treatment planning systems.

TPS Name	Latest Version	Institution	Calculation Code	Facilities Used	Update
NCTPlan	MacNCTPlan, 2002	Harvard/MIT	MCNP	MITR, RA6	No
SERA	SERA-1C1, 2005	INEEL/MSU	seraMC	KUR, FiR 1, *etc.*	No
JCDS	JCDS-FX, 2011	KURRI	MCNP/ PHITS	JRR-4	No
THORplan	THORplan4, 2018	National Tsing Hua University	MCNP	THOR	Yes
SACRA Planning	NeuCure®, 2020	SHI	PHITS	Accelerator-based	Yes
Tsukuba-Plan	—	Tsukuba University	PHITS	Accelerator-based	Yes
—	—	CICS	PHITS	Accelerator-based	Yes
—	—	NTI	—	Accelerator-based	Yes
NeuMANTA	NeuMANTA®, 2022	NeuBoron	COMPASS	Accelerator-based	Yes

(1) *Obtaining medical image data of patients*

For dose assessment using a TPS, medical image (CT, MRI) data of the patient are first acquired as a basis for creating a computational model. Since the Monte Carlo method is used for dose calculation in the treatment planning of BNCT, it takes more time to calculate the dose compared to conventional X-ray therapy, *etc.*, so although it also depends on the specifications of the computer, it is best to obtain medical image data as early as possible. Generally, CT images are used for treatment planning, but for a system having the function of data fusion using a plurality of medical images, MRI and PET image data can also be acquired. For imaging conditions of CT images, the slice interval is generally 2 mm to 5 mm. The narrower the slice interval, the more accurate the patient model can be formed.

(2) *Material definition*

Based on imported CT data (or MRI data), first set up regions for each material. Here, since the behavior of the radiation during X-ray therapy depends on the electron density, the material can in principle be precisely defined using the CT value of each CT pixel. However, since the Monte Carlo method is used in the dose assessment of BNCT, it is necessary to define the composition information for each tissue, which is different from the material definition of the X-ray TPS. Usually in the case of BNCT, the behavior of neutrons depends on the density of hydrogen atoms, so the material is divided into regions according to the density of hydrogen atoms. In general, the behavior of neutrons can be calculated roughly in three types: air, soft tissue, and bone. To perform transport calculations with higher accuracy, it is necessary to further segment tissues with different hydrogen densities (such as muscle, fat, *etc.*) and define materials.

For the composition information of each type of tissue, one could consider using ICRU-46 as a reference.

(3) *Region of interest settings*

After the definition of the material area, set the ROI (region of interest) for the area where dose assessment is to be performed. This ROI includes the tumor. For example, in the treatment of malignant brain tumors, tumorous tissue, brain, skin, *etc.*, can be defined as ROI. Herein, in the case of malignant brain tumors, the ROI area is considered to include both the gross tumor volume (GTV) and the clinical target volume (CTV). GTV is clearly visible to the naked eye and shows the position and extent of gross tumor, whereas the CTV, also defined as the treatment site, contains the GTV plus a margin of microscopic infiltration of the tumor. To achieve successful treatment, the CTV must be adequately treated. It is challenging to accurately define the CTV for an individual patient because the normal tissue and cancer cells are likely to mix in the areas of the tumor spread. Therefore, in this region, both normal tissue (brain) and tumor dose assessments must be performed.

(4) *Setting of irradiation conditions*
Irradiation conditions are set on the 3D model of the patient for which material definition and ROI have been set. Typically, irradiation conditions include: (a) the shape and size of the neutron beam aperture, (b) the distance from the beam aperture to the patient, and (c) the incidence range and angle of the neutron beam relative to the patient model. In addition, to achieve dose calculations, the average boron concentration (ppm) in each tissue is defined. In the case of an irradiation apparatus capable of changing the quality of the neutron beam to be irradiated, it is necessary to set the neutron spectrum and intensity of the beam used for treatment.

(5) *Generate computational models*
The calculation model is generated based on the 3D model of the patient with the material definition and irradiation conditions set. In general, Monte Carlo computations use a modeling method called the voxel method. Voxel models used for Monte Carlo calculations are often converted to "rough" geometric computational models for efficient computation of CT pixel data used to create a 3D model of the patient. For example, by "rounding" four pixels into a voxel, the phantom of each slice becomes a reduced model. Typically, when four pixels are combined into one, the texture composition of the four pixels is averaged and rounded.

In addition, for the 3D computational model of the patient, the source information of the irradiated neutron beam (energy spectrum of neutrons and photons, angular distribution, *etc.*) and the geometric information of the equipment (beam irradiation aperture, surrounding shielding, *etc.*) are combined to complete the computational model.

(6) *Dose distribution calculation*
Using the computational model, a Monte Carlo-based transport calculation is implemented. In the dose calculation, neutron and photon transport calculations are performed, and each absorbed dose at each

point (each voxel) within the patient model is calculated. In transport calculations, Monte Carlo calculation programs such as MCNP and PHITS are used in conjunction with a nuclear database that stores information such as nuclear reaction cross-sections between elements and neutrons/photons. Nuclear databases include ENDF/B in the U.S. and JENDL in Japan. By using the Kerma factor stored in the respective nuclear databases, the absorbed dose can be calculated automatically by multiplying the Kerma factor corresponding to the neutron/photon energy spectrum at each point.

(7) Analysis of calculation results
The results are organized and output as data that can be used for treatment planning. Here, since the calculation is performed with a rough phantom in the computational model, each pixel of the original CT is usually interpolated and assigned the calculation result. Next, the calculation results are assigned to each ROI, and the maximum, minimum, and average doses of each are calculated. In addition, the dose volume histogram of each ROI is calculated. Even the neutron distribution, photon distribution, and dose distribution (each absorbed dose, and equivalent dose) on each slice of CT and MRI medical images are shown for easy understanding.

5.4 Treatment Process

A basic flow chart for BNCT treatment process is shown in Figure 5.27. For a clinical facility specialized for BNCT, applications will be received from patients with a variety of conditions and indications. First of all, pre-BNCT flow shows the preparation work that needs to be done before the treatment. Before registration, it is necessary to judge whether BNCT is possible based on the physical condition of the patient and the treatment received so far. If possible, a medical examination and various tests will be performed by a specialist to determine the final applicability. After registration, the patient undergoes a PET scan with ^{18}F-BPA to determine the tumor-to-normal tissue ratio of ^{10}B concentration, followed by CT and MRI. Accordingly, the treatment planning will be done, and the dose prescription completed.

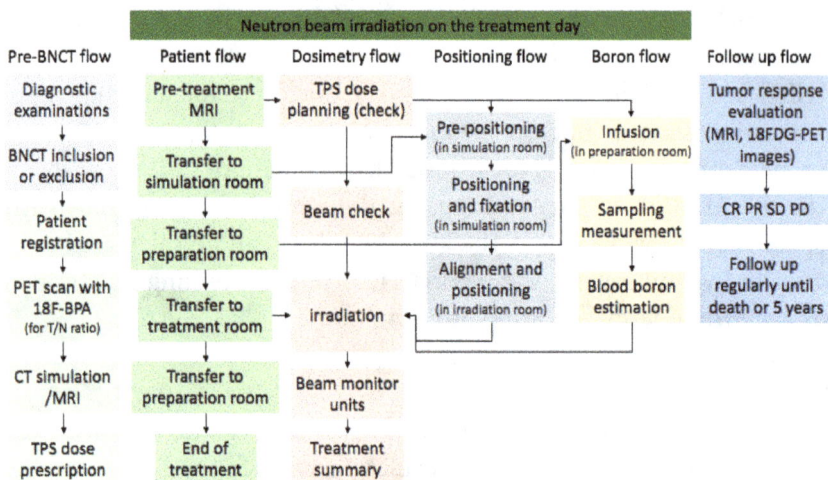

Pre-BNCT flow	Patient flow	Dosimetry flow	Positioning flow	Boron flow	Follow up flow

Figure 5.27 Basic flow chart of the BNCT treatment process.

On the day of treatment, the patient receives neutron irradiation. The patient needs to undergo an MRI scan for TPS dose planning check first. In the meantime, the staff carry out the beam checking work, such as operating the neutron source, executing a QC/QA program for Au/Cu foil activation, paired ionization chambers, fission chamber neutron monitors, and ICP-AES for boron concentration measurement. Neutron beam irradiation parameters including patient collimation, patient alignment and positioning, prescription dose, neutron source power and irradiation time will also be determined. The patient is then moved to the simulation room for positioning and fixation. Afterwards, patient is transferred to the preparation room and the BPA infusion is started. The first and second blood samples will be collected for ^{10}B concentration determination 1 and 2 hours after the start of the BPA infusion, respectively. After that, the infusion flow will be halved. Then the patient is moved to the treatment room for quick alignment and positioning. Before the treatment begins, the staff in the BNCT control room will input the operation parameters into the online monitoring system, include the prescription dose, background and boron dose rate, boron concentration in blood, *etc.*, and call the neutron source to start up to the specified power and initiate the irradiation. Typically, the irradiation time is 20 to 30 minutes. After irradiation, the patient is transferred back to the preparation room. The nurse will take a third blood sample and stop the BPA infusion. Meanwhile, the patient surface dose rate and activation will be measured by using a γ ray dosimeter and a high-purity germanium detector, respectively. At the same time, a treatment summary will be prepared.

After neutron irradiation therapy, according to MRI and [18]FDG-PET images, tumor response evaluation will be estimated based on criteria among CR (complete response), PR (partial response), SD (stable disease), and PD (progressive disease) in RECIST (Response Evaluation Criteria in Solid Tumors). After treatment, patients will be followed regularly for five years or until death [45].

References

1. Levin, V. and Andreo, P. (Eds.) (2001). *Current Status of Neutron Capture Therapy, IAEA-TECDOC-1223.* International Atomic Energy Agency.
2. Brown, D. A., *et al.* (2018). ENDF/B-VIII.0: The 8th major release of the nuclear reaction data library with CIELO-project cross sections, new standards and thermal scattering data. *Nucl. Data Sheets* **148**, 1–142.
3. Chadwick, J. (1932). Possible existence of a neutron. *Nature* **129**, 312.
4. Chadwick, J. (1932). The existence of a neutron. *Proc. R. Soc. Lond. A* **136**, 692–708.
5. Chadwick, J. and Goldhaber, M. (1934). A 'nuclear photo-effect': Disintegration of the diplon by γ-rays. *Nature* **134**, 237–238.
6. Chadwick J. and Goldhaber, M. (1935). Disintegration by slow neutron. *Nature* **135**, 65.
7. Taylor, H. and Goldhaber, M. (1935). Detection of nuclear disintegration in a photographic emulsion. *Nature* **135**, 341.
8. Burcham, W. E. and Goldhaber, M. (1936). The disintegration of nitrogen by slow neutrons. *Math. Proc. Camb. Philos. Soc.* **32**, 632–636.
9. Crease, R. P. and Goldhaber, A. S. (2012). *A Biographical Memoir of Maurice Goldharber (1911–2011).* National Academy of Sciences.
10. Locher, G. L. (1936). Biological effects and therapeutic possibilities of neutrons. *Am. J. Roentgenol. Radium Ther.* **36**, 1–13.
11. Kruger, P. G. (1940). Some biological effects of nuclear disintegration products on neoplastic tissue. *Proc. Natl. Acad. Sci.* **26**, 181–192.
12. Sweet, W. H. and Javid, M. (1951). The possible use of slow neutrons plus boron10 in therapy of intracranial tumors. *Trans. Am. Neurol. Assoc.* **56**, 60–63.

13. Sweet, W. H. (1951). The uses of nuclear disintegration in the diagnosis and treatment of brain tumor. *N. Engl. J. Med.* **245**, 875–878.

14. Farr, L. E., Sweet, W. H., Robertson, J. S., Foster, C. G., Locksley, H. B., Sutherland, D. L., *et al.* (1954). Neutron capture therapy with boron in the treatment of glioblastoma multiforme. *Am. J. Roentgenol. Radium Ther. Nucl. Med.* **71**, 279–293.

15. Farr, L. E., Sweet, W. H., Locksley, H. B. and Robertson, J. S. (1954). Neutron capture therapy of gliomas using boron. *Trans. Am. Neurol. Assoc.* **13**, 110–113.

16. Farr, L. E., Robertson, J. S. and Stickley, E. (1954). Physics and physiology of neutron-capture therapy. *Proc. Natl. Acad. Sci.* **40**, 1087–1093.

17. Slatkin, D. N. (1991). A history of boron neutron capture therapy of brain tumours. *Brain* **114**, 1609–1629.

18. Slatkin, D. N., Javid, M. J., Joel, D. D., Kalef-Ezra, J. A., Ma, R., Feinendegen, L. E. *et al.* (2017). A history of 20th-century boron neutron capture therapy. *J. Neurol. Neurobiol.* **3**, 2.

19. Fairchild, R. G. (1965). Development and dosimetry of an 'epithermal' neutron beam for possible use in neutron capture therapy I. 'Epithermal' neutron beam development. *Phys. Med. Biol.* **10**, 491–504.

20. Fairchild, R. G., Kalef-Ezra, J., Saraf, S. K., Fiarman, S., Ramsey, E., Wielopolski, L., *et al.* (1990). Installation and testing of an optimized epithermal neutron beam at the Brookhaven Medical Research Reactor (BMRR). *Basic Life Sci.* **54**, 185–199.

21 Choi, J. R., Clement, S. D., Harling, O. K. and Zamenhorf, R. O. (1990). Neutron capture therapy beams at the MIT research reactor. *Basic Life Sci.* **54**, 201–218.

22. Miller, H. C., Miller, N. E. and Muetterties, E. L. (1963). Synthesis of polyhedral boranes. *J. Am. Chem. Soc.* **85**, 3885–3886.

23. Knoth, W. H., Sauer, J. C., England, D. C., Hertler, W. R. and Muetterties, E. L. (1964). Chemistry of borons. XIX. Derivative chemistry of $B_{10}H_{10}^{-2}$ and $B_{12}H_{12}^{-2}$. *J. Am. Chem. Soc.* **86**, 3973–3983.

24. Soloway, A. H., Hatanaka, H. and Davis, M. A. (1967). Penetration of brain and brain tumor. VII. Tumor-binding sulfhydryl boron compounds. *J. Med. Chem.* **10**, 714–717.

25. Hatanaka, H. (1990). Clinical results of boron neutron capture therapy. *Basic Life Sci.* **54**, 15–21.

26. Sirai, E., Takahashi, H., Issiki, M., Arigane, K., Iwaya, M., Hatanaka, H., *et al.* (1992). Clinical Experience of BNCT for Brain Tumours at JAERI. In: Allen, B. J., Moore D. E. and Harrington, B. V. (Eds.), *Progress in Neutron Capture Therapy for Cancer*, Springer, pp. 569–576.

27. Nakagawa, Y. and Hatanaka, H. (1997). Boron neutron capture therapy. Clinical brain tumor studies. *J. Neurooncol.* **33**, 105–115.

28. Mishima, Y., Ichihashi, M., Hatta, S., Honda, C., Yamamura, K., Nakagawa, T., *et al.* (1989). First human clinical trial of melanoma neutron capture. Diagnosis and therapy. *Strahlenther. Onkol.* **165**, 251–254.
29. Mishima, Y., Ichihashi, M., Hatta, S., Honda, C., Sasase, A., Yamamura, K., *et al.* (1989). Selective thermal neutron capture therapy and diagnosis of malignant melanoma: from basic studies to first clinical treatment. *Basic Life Sci.* **50**, 251–260.
30. Kobayashi, T., Sakurai, Y., Kanda, K., Fujita, Y. and Ono, K. (2000). The remodeling and basic characteristics of the heavy water neutron irradiation facility of the Kyoto University Research Reactor, mainly for neutron capture therapy. *Nucl. Technol.* **131**, 354–378.
31. Sakurai, Y., Tanaka, H., Takata, T., Fujimoto, N., Suzuki, M., Masunaga, S., *et al.* (2015). Advances in boron neutron capture therapy (BNCT) at Kyoto University — From reactor-based BNCT to accelerator-based BNCT. *J. Korean Phys. Soc.* **67**, 76–81.
32. Nakai, K., Yamamoto, T., Kumada, H. and Matsumura, A. (2014). Boron neutron capture therapy for glioblastoma: a phase-I/II clinical trial at JRR-4. *Eur. Assoc. NeuroOncol. Mag.* **4**, 116–123.
33 Yoshiya, T., Kazuyoshi, Y., Naohiko, H., Hiroaki, K. and Yoji, H. (2001). JRR-4 medical irradiation facility. *JAERI-Conf 2001–017.* 352–356. :2001/11
34. Chanana, A. D., Capala, J., Chadha, M., Coderre, J. A., Diaz, A. Z., Elowitz, E. H., *et al.* (1999). Boron neutron capture therapy for glioblastoma multiforme: interim results from the phase I/II dose-escalation studies. *Neurosurgery* **44**, 1182–1192.
35. Busse, P. M., Harling, O. K., Palmer, M. R., Kiger III, W. S., Kaplan, J., Kaplan, I., *et al.* (2003). A critical examination of the results from the Harvard-MIT NCT program phase I clinical trial of neutron capture therapy for intracranial disease. *J. Neurooncol.* **62**, 111–121.
36. Moss, R. L., Stecher-Rasmussen, F., Ravensverg, K., Constantine, G. and Watkins, P. (1992). Design, Construction and Installation of an Epithermal Neutron Beam for BNCT at the High Flux Reactor Petten. In: Allen, B. J., Moore, D. E. and Harrington, B.V. (Eds.), *Progress in Neutron Capture Therapy for Cancer*, Springer, pp. 63–66.
37. Auterinen, I., Hiismäki, P., Kotiluoto, P., Rosenberg, R. J., Salmenhaara, S., Seppälä, T., *et al.* (2001). Metamorphosis of a 35-Year-Old TRIGA Reactor into a Modern BNCT Facility. In: Hawthorne, M. F., Shelly, K. and Wiersema, R. J. (Eds.), *Frontiers in Neutron Capture Therapy*, Springer, pp. 267–275.
38. Henriksson, R., Capala, J., Michanek, A., Lindahl, S. A., Salford, L. G., Franzén, E., *et al.* (2008). Boron neutron capture therapy (BNCT) for glioblastoma multiforme: a phase II study evaluating a prolonged high-dose of boronophenylalanine (BPA). *Radiother. Oncol.* **88**, 183–191.
39. Dbalý, V., Tovaryš, F., Honova, H., Petruželka, L., Prokes, K., Burian, J., *et al.* (2002). Contemporary state of neutron capture therapy in Czech Republich (Part 2). *Čes. Slov. Neurol. Neurochir.* **66**, 60–63.

40. Menéndez, P. R., Roth, B. M. C., Pereira, M. D., Casal, M. R., Gonzalez, D S., Feld, J. B., *et al.* (2009). BNCT for skin melanoma in extremities: updated Argentine clinical results. *Appl. Radiat. Isot.* **67**, S50–53.

41. Wang, L. W., Hsueh Liu, Y. W., Chou F. I. and Jiang, S. H. (2018). Clinical trials for treating recurrent head and neck cancer with boron neutron capture therapy using the Tsing-Hua open pool reactor. *Cancer Commun.* **38**, 37.

42. Yong, Z., Song, Z., Zhou, Y., Liu, T., Zhang, Z., Zhao, Y., *et al.* (2016). Boron neutron capture therapy for malignant melanoma: first clinical case report in China. *Chin. J. Cancer Res.* **28**, 634–640.

43. Kankaanranta, L., Seppälä, T., Kallio, M., Karila, J., Aschan, C., Serén, T., *et al.* (2000). First clinical results on the Finnish study on BPA-mediated BNCT in glioblastoma. In: *Program & Abstracts of 9th International Symposium on Neutron Capture Therapy for Cancer*, Osaka, Japan.

44. Barth, R. F., Vicente, M. G., Harling, O. K., Kiger III, W. S., Riley, K. J., Binns, P. J., *et al.* (2012). Current status of boron neutron capture therapy of high-grade gliomas and recurrent head and neck cancer. *Radiat. Oncol.* **7**, 146.

45. Jiang, S. H., Hsueh Liu, Y. W., Chou, F. I., Liu, H. M., Peir, J. J., Liu, Y. H., *et al.* (2020). The overview and prospects of BNCT facility at Tsing Hua open-pool reactor. *Appl. Radiat. Isot.* **161**, 109143.

46. Moss, R. L. (2014). Critical review, with an optimistic outlook, on boron neutron capture therapy (BNCT). *Appl. Radiat. Isot.* **88**, 2–11.

47. Nigg, D. W. (Ed.) (1994). *Proceedings of the First International Workshop on Accelerator-Based Neutron Sources for Boron Neutron Capture Therapy.* CONF-940976. Idaho National Engineering Laboratory, USA.

48. Nigg, D. W. (2006). Neutron Sources and Applications in Radiotherapy — A Brief History and Current Trends. In: *12th International Symposium on Neutron Capture Therapy*, Takamatsu, Japan.

49. Blue, T. E. and Yanch, J. C. (2003). Accelerator-based epithermal neutron sources for boron neutron capture therapy of brain tumors. *J. Neuro-Oncol.* **62**, 19–31.

50. Kreiner, A. J. (2012). Accelerator-Based BNCT. In: Sauerwein, W. A. G., Witting, A., Moss, R. and Nakagawa, Y. (Eds.), *Neutron Capture Therapy: Principles and Applications*, Springer, pp. 41–54.

51. Kreiner, A. J., Bergueiro, J., Cartelli, D., Baldo, M., Castell, W., Asoia, J. G., *et al.* (2016). Present status of accelerator-based BNCT. *Rep. Pract. Oncol. Radiother.* **21**, 95–101.

52. Cartelli, D. E., Capoulat, M. E., Baldo, M., Suarez Sandín, J. C., Igarzabal, M., Del Grosso, M. F., *et al.* (2020). Status of low-energy accelerator-based BNCT worldwide and in Argentina. *Appl. Radiat. Isot.* **166**, 109315.

53. Tanaka, H., Sakurai, Y., Suzuki, M., Masunaga, S., Kinashi, Y., Kashino, G., *et al.* (2009). Characteristics comparison between a cyclotron-based neutron source and KUR-HWNIF for boron neutron capture therapy. *Nucl. Instrum. Methods Phys. Res. B.* **267**, 1970–1977.

54. Tanaka, H. (2021). Current status of accelerator-based boron neutron capture therapy (BNCT) (in Japanese). *Igaku Butsuri.* **41**, 117–121.
55. Porra, L., Seppälä, T., Wendland, L., Revitzer, H., Joensuu, H., Eide, P., *et al.* (2022). Accelerator-based boron neutron capture therapy facility at the Helsinki University Hospital. *Acta Oncol.* **61**, 269–273.
56. Porras, I., Praena, J., Arias de Saavedra, F., Pedrosa-Rivera, M., Torres-Sanchez, P., Sabariego, M. P., *et al.* (2020). BNCT research activities at the Granada group and the project NeMeSis: Neutrons for medicine and sciences, towards an accelerator-based facility for new BNCT therapies, medical isotope production and other scientific neutron applications. *Appl. Radiat. Isot.* **165**, 109247.
57. Harling, O. K. and Riley, K. J. (2012). Fission Reactor-Based Irradiation Facilities for Neutron Capture Therapy. In: Sauerwein, W., Wittig, A., Moss, R. and Nakagawa, H. (Eds.), *Neutron Capture Therapy: Principles and Applications,* Springer, pp. 19–40.
58. Harling, O. K. (2009). Fission reactor based epithermal neutron irradiation facilities for routine clinical application in BNCT — Hatanaka memorial lecture. *Appl. Radiat. Isot.* **67**, S7–S11.
59. Harling, O. K. and Riley, K. J. (2003). Fission reactor neutron sources for neutron capture therapy — a critical review. *J. Neuro-Oncol.* **62**, 7–17.
60. Rief, H., Van Heusden, R. and Perlini, G. Generating Epithermal Neutron Beams for Neutron Capture Therapy in Small Reactors. In: Soloway, A. H., Barth, R. F. and Carpenter, D. E. (Eds.), *Advances in Neutron Capture Therapy*, Springer, pp. 85–88.
61. Harling, O. K., Riley, K. J., Newton, T. H., Wilson, B. A., Bernard, J. A., Hu, L. W., *et al.* (2002). The fission converter-based epithermal neutron irradiation facility at the Massachusetts Institute of Technology reactor. *Nucl. Sci. Eng.* **140**, 223–240.
62. Liu, H. B., Brugger, R. M., Rorer, D. C., Tichler, P. R. and Hu, J. P. (1994). Design of a high-flux epithermal neutron beam using 235U fission plates at the Brookhaven Medical Research Reactor. *Med. Phys.* **21**, 1627–1631.
63. Liu, H. B., Razvi, J., Rucker, R., Cerbone, R., Merrill, M., Whittemore, W., *et al.* (2001). TRIGA Fuel Based Converter Assembly Design for a Dual-Mode Neutron Beam System at the McClellan Nuclear Radiation Center. In: Hawthorne, M. F., Shelly, K. and Wiersema, R. J. (Eds.), *Frontiers in Neutron Capture Therapy*, Springer, pp. 295–300.
64. Ke, G. T., Sun, Z. Y., Shen, F., Liu, T. C., Li, Y. G. and Zhou, Y. M. (2009). The study of physics and thermal characteristics for in-hospital neutron irradiator (IHNI). *Appl. Radiat. Isot.* **67**, S234–S237.
65. Sauerwein, W. and Moss, R. L. (Eds.) (2013). *Requirements for Boron Neutron Capture Therapy (BNCT) at a Nuclear Research Reactor.* Publications Office, Joint Research Centre, Institute for Energy and Transport.
66. Virtual Technical Meeting on Advances in Boron Neutron Capture Therapy. (2020). https://nucleus.iaea.org/sites/accelerators/TMBNCT/SitePages/Home%202020.aspx.

67. Daquino, G. G. and Voorbraak, W. P. (2009). *A Review of the Recommendations for the Physical Dosimetry of Boron Neutron Capture Therapy (BNCT)*. Publications Office, Joint Research Centre, Institute for Energy and Transport.

68. Sessler, A. and Wilson, E. (2007). *Engines of Discovery: A Century of Particle Accelerators*. World Scientific.

69. Tanaka, H., Sakurai, Y., Suzuki, M., Takata, T., Masunaga, S., Kinashi, Y., *et al.* (2009). Improvement of dose distribution in phantom by using epithermal neutron source based on the Be(p,n) reaction using a 30 MeV proton cyclotron accelerator. *Appl. Radiat. Isot.* **67**, S258–S261.

70. Suzuki, M., Tanaka, H., Sakurai, Y., Kashino, G., Yong, L., Masunaga, S., *et al.* (2009). Impact of accelerator-based boron neutron therapy (AB-BNCT) on the treatment of multiple liver tumors and malignant pleural mesothelioma. *Radiother. Oncol.* **92**, 89–95.

71. Tanaka, H., Sakurai, Y., Suzuki, M., Masunaga, S., Mitsumoto, T., Fujita, K., *et al.* (2011). Experimental verification of beam characteristics for cyclotron-based epithermal neutron source (C-BENS). *Appl. Radiat. Isot.* **69**, 1642–1645.

72. Kato, T., Hirose, K., Tanaka, H., Mitsumoto, T., Motoyanagi, T., Arai, K., *et al.* (2020). Design and construction of an accelerator-based boron neutron capture therapy (AB-BNCT) facility with multiple treatment rooms at the Southern Tohoku BNCT Research Center. *Appl. Radiat. Isot.* **156**, 108961.

73. Hirose, K., Konno, A., Hiratsuka, J., Yoshimoto, S., Kato, T., Ono, K., *et al.* (2021). Boron neutron capture therapy using cyclotron-based epithermal neutron source and borofalan (^{10}B) for recurrent or locally advanced head and neck cancer (JHN002): An open-label phase II trial. *Radiother. Oncol.* **155**, 182–187.

74. Kawabata, S., Suzuki, M., Hirose, K., Tanaka, H., Kato, T., Goto, H., *et al.* (2021). Accelerator-based BNCT for patients with recurrent glioblastoma: a multicenter phase II study. *Neurooncol. Adv.* **3**, 1–9.

75. Mitsumoto, T., Yajima, S., Tsutsui, H., Ogasawara, T., Fujita, K., Tanaka, H., *et al.* (2013). Cyclotron-based neutron source for BNCT. *AIP Conf. Proc.* **1525**, 319.

76. Allen, D. A. and Beynon, T. D. (1995). A design study for an accelerator-based epithermal neutron beam for BNCT. *Phys. Med. Biol.* **40**, 807–821.

77. Allen, D. A., Beynon, T. D. and Green, S. (1999). Design for an accelerator-based orthogonal epithermal neutron beam for boron neutron capture therapy. *Med. Phys.* **26**, 71–76.

78. Forton, E., Stichelbaut, F., Cambriani, A., Kleeven, W., Ahlback, J. and Jongen, Y. (2009). Overview of the IBA accelerator-based BNCT system. *Appl. Radiat. Isot.* **67**, S262–S265.

79. Kiyanagi, Y., Tsuchida, K., Uritani, A., Kawabata, Y., Yamazaki, A., Menjoh, Y., *et al.* (2014). Project of electrostatic accelerator-based BNCT system in Nagoya University. In: *Proceedings of the 11th Annual Meeting of Particle Accelerator Society of Japan*, Aomori, Japan.

80. Watanabe, K., Yoshihashi, S., Ishikawa, A., Honda, S., Yamazaki, A., Tsurita, Y., et al. (2021). First experimental verification of the neutron field of Nagoya University Accelerator-driven neutron source for boron neutron capture therapy. *Appl. Radiat. Isot.* **168**, 109553.
81. Yanch, J. C., Shefer, R. E., Klinkowstein, R. E., Howard, W. B., Song, H., Blackburn, B., et al. (1997). Research in boron neutron capture therapy at MIT LABA. *AIP Conf. Proc.* **392**, 1281.
82. Shefer, R. E., Klinkowstein, R. E. and Yanch, J. C. (1997). A high current electrostatic accelerator for boron neutron capture therapy. In: *Proc. SPIE 2867, International Conference Neutrons in Research and Industry,* Crete, Greece.
83. Bayanov, B., Belov, V., Bender, E., Bokhovko, M. V., Dimov, G. I., Kononov, V. N., et al. (1998). Accelerator based neutron sources for the neutron-capture and fast neutron therapy at hospital. *Nucl. Instrum. Methods Phys. Res. A* **413**, 397–426.
84. Ivanov, A. A., Sanin, A., Belchenko, Y., Gusev, I., Emelev, I., Rashchenko, V., et al. (2021). Recent achievements in studies of negative beam formation and acceleration in the tandem accelerator at Budker Institute. *AIP Conf. Proc.* **2373**, 070002.
85. Dymova, M. A., Taskaev, S. Y., Richter, V. A. and Kuligina, E. V. (2020). Boron neutron capture therapy: Current status and future perspectives. *Cancer Commun.* **40**, 406–421.
86. Kwan, J. W., Anderson, O. A., Reginato, L. L., Vella, M. C. and Yu, S. S. (1994). Electrostatic quadrupole DC accelerators for BNCT applications, LBL-35540. In: *International Workshop on Accelerator-Based Neutron Sources for Boron Neutron Capture Therapy,* Wyoming, USA.
87. Kwan, J. W., Ackerman, G. D., Chan, C. F., Cooper, W. S., de Vries, G. J., Steele, W. F., et al. (1995). Acceleration of 100 mA of H — in a single channel electrostatic quadrupole accelerator. *Rev. Sci. Instrum.* **66**, 3864.
88. Ludewigt, B. A., Chu, W. T., Donahue, R. J., Kwan, J., Phillips, T. J., Reginato, L. L., et al. (1997). An epithermal neutron source for BNCT based on an ESQ-accelerator, LBNL-40642. In: *American Nuclear Society (ANS) Winter Meeting,* New Mexico, USA.
89. Kreiner, A. J., Kwan, J. W., Burlón, A. A., Di Paolo, H., Henestroza, E., Minsky, D. M., et al. (2007). A tandem-ESQ for accelerator-based boron neutron capture therapy. *Nucl. Instrum. Methods B* **261**, 751–754.
90. Wangler, T. P., Sovall, J. E., Bhatia, T. S., Wang, C. K., Blue, T. E. and Gahbauer, R. A. (1989). Conceptual design of an RFQ accelerator-based neutron source for boron neutron-capture therapy. In: *Proceedings of the 1989 IEEE Particle Accelerator Conference, 'Accelerator Science and Technology',* Illinois, USA.
91. Swenson, D. A. (1999). Compact, inexpensive, epithermal neutron source for BNCT. *AIP Conf. Proc.* **475**, 1037.
92. Swenson, D. (2015). RFI-based ion linac systems. *Physics Procedia.* **66**, 177–179.

93. Pisent, A., Fagotti, E., Lamanna, G. V. and Mathot, S. (2004). The Trasco-Spes RFQ. In: *Proceedings of the LINAC 2004 Conference*, Lübeck, Germany.
94. Fujii, R., Imahori, Y., Nakakmura, M., Takada, M., Kamada, S., Hamano, T., *et al.* (2012). Lithium target for accelerator based BNCT neutron source: Influence by the proton irradiation on lithium. *AIP Conf. Proc.* **1509**, 162–170.
95. The ultimate method of treating intractable cancer is "BNCT (Boron Neutron Capture Therapy)". (2019). https://www.cics.jp/page/english.html.
96. Chen, J. Y., Tong, J. F., Hu, Z. L., Han, X. F., Tang, B., Yu, Q., *et al.* (2022). Evaluation of neutron beam characteristics for D-BNCT01 facility. *Nucl. Sci. Tech.* **33**, 12.
97. Kumada, H., Matsumura, A., Sakurai, H., Sakae, T., Yoshioka, M., Kobayashi, H., *et al.* (2014). Project for the development of the linac based NCT facility in University of Tsukuba. *Appl. Radiat. Isot.* **88**, 211–215.
98. Kumada, H., Takada, K., Tanaka, S., Matsumoto, Y., Naito, F., Kur Ihara, T., *et al.* (2020). Evaluation of the characteristics of the neutron beam of a linac-based neutron source for boron neutron capture therapy. *Appl. Radiat. Isot.* **165**, 109246.
99. Nakamura, S., Igaki, H., Ito, M., *et al.* (2019). Characterization of the relationship between neutron production and thermal load on a target material in an accelerator-based boron neutron capture therapy system employing a solid-state Li target. *PLoS ONE* **14**(11), e0225587.
100. Yoshioka, M. (2016). Review of accelerator-based boron neutron capture therapy machines. In: *Proceedings of IPAC2016*, Busan, Korea.

Index

www.ingramcontent.com/pod-product-compliance
Lightning Source LLC
Chambersburg PA
CBHW050558190326
41458CB00007B/2086